Policy and Place: General Medi

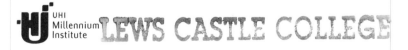

Also by Graham Moon:

Health, Disease and Society (with Kelvyn Jones), Routledge

Society and Health (edited with Rosemary Gillespie), Routledge

Epidemiology: an introduction (with Myles Gould and colleagues), Open
  University Press

Urban Policy in Britain (with Rob Atkinson), Macmillan

Also by Nancy North:

Perspectives in Health (with Yvonne Bradshaw), Macmillan

Policy and Place
General Medical Practice in the UK

Graham Moon
and
Nancy North

First Published 2000 by
MACMILLAN PRESS LTD
Houndmills, Basingstoke, Hampshire RG21 6XS
and London
Companies and representatives
throughout the world

ISBN 0–333–73039–9 paperback

A catalogue record for this book is available
from the British Library.

This book is printed on paper suitable for recycling and
made from fully managed and sustained forest sources.

10 9   8   7   6   5   4   3   2   1
09 08 07 06 05 04 03 02 01 00

Editing and origination by
Aardvark Editorial, Mendham, Suffolk

Printed in Malaysia

To Liz Twigg and Derek North

Contents

List of Figures

List of Tables

Acknowledgements

To Ian Kendall and Rudolf Klein for their constructive criticism of two of the chapters; the Department of Health, the NHS Management Executive, the Welsh Office, the Scottish Executive and the Department of Health and Social Services, Northern Ireland, for patiently clarifying certain details; Janet Hopton, Brenda Poulton, Margaret Smith, the General Medical Council, the Medical Defence Union and the Scottish Consumer Council for information graciously given; Roisin Gwyer for assistance in chasing down references; and finally Richenda Milton-Thompson at the publishers for her forbearance.

1

Introduction

> We take our GPs for granted. It is not just that we expect them to be there on tap, reliable, proficient, sympathetic, free... We also assume that there is something right and natural about the very existence of the family doctor as first port of call, providing a full range of primary care and giving us access to specialists and hospitals. (Porter 1999, reviewing Loudon *et al.* 1998)

The vast majority of the UK population are registered with a general medical practice from which they expect (and receive) care and treatment for general health problems and onward referral for more specialist attention. Most people who fall ill and decide to seek medical care therefore first see a general practitioner (GP). A GP will usually see an expectant mother during pregnancy, sustained absence from work will require authentication by a GP, and many deaths are certified by GPs. The GP controls access to further care, most notably hospital treatment, and is central to the provision of continuity of care for people discharged from hospital. This book examines policy and its current implementation with regard to general medical practice, a service that can justly be portrayed as a therapeutic cornerstone of the UK National Health Service (NHS).

Although it was not always so, the therapeutic salience of general medical practice is now matched by a political importance. General practice provides a setting for the delivery of primary care, and primary care is promoted nationally and internationally as the key means of enhancing health status. Within the UK context, it was with a White Paper on primary care that the Conservative Party's programme of reform for the NHS was launched in the late 1980s. In that reform programme, general practice was the basis of arguably the most innovative development – the general practice fundholding initiative. The election of a New Labour government in 1997 saw an extension of this political and policy profile. The creation of primary care groups in England, and their equivalents in Wales, Scotland and Northern Ireland, has placed general practices and GPs at the political core of the NHS.

The aim of this book is to present a sympathetic yet critical analysis of general practice. The intention is to examine how it has come to occupy the position that it now holds within the NHS, evaluate the diverse impacts that health care reform has had on the provision and delivery of general medical services, and assess key challenges that are now being faced. To address this task, the book will draw on both our own research and an original synthesis and evaluation of the work of others. This introductory chapter provides a scene-setting. It begins with a consideration of NHS general practice. This elaborates on the themes introduced in the first paragraph and defines the subject matter of the book – GPs and general practice. It considers the characteristics of the GP population as well as what they do and whether any other country can truly be said to have a similar sort of service. The second part of the chapter presents the evidence for the increasing political importance of general practice. This chronology of reform and review provides an important underpinning framework for much of the rest of the book. A short discussion of the rationale for the book and a summary of its structure conclude the chapter.

NHS General Practice

For readers unfamiliar with the UK NHS, it is perhaps necessary to begin with a broad descriptive summary of what general practice is and what GPs do. In essence, GPs and general practice are about the diagnosis and treatment of ill-health without any limitation on the age or sex of the patient or any restriction regarding the types of illness that are being presented. General practice is therefore first and fundamentally about general medicine. The subject matter of consultations can cover the full gamut of human ill-health, the physical and the psychosocial, the obvious and the obscure, the life-threatening and the merely discomforting. This widely ranging subject matter demands a particular form of training and particular skills. The emphasis has to be on the breadth of possibilities rather than on detailed issues, as with more traditional medical specialisations. In fact, the defining characteristic of the specialism of general practice is its very generality.

A second characteristic of general practice, which should be noted at the outset, is its status as the initial point of contact with the NHS for individuals who decide to seek biomedical health care for a health problem. Around 90 per cent of illness is managed outside hospitals (Baggott 1994). When people speak of seeing a doctor, they will usually be referring to a GP. If they are not and they are talking of an appointment with a hospital clinician, they will have accessed that specialist service via a referral from a GP. GPs thus provide first-line care and are the people who make onward referrals to hospital care. In other words, they provide primary care and are the gate-keepers of secondary care. In the context of the UK NHS, the vast majority of this care is also free, at least as far as the consultation between the GP and patient is concerned. The subsequent meeting with the pharmacist to exchange a prescription for a regime of drug treatment will, in many cases, necessitate a small cash transaction, and the whole system is, of course, paid for by tax.

A third generalisation relates to the nature of the relationship between the GP and the patient. In theory, people are free to choose their own GP and to change their GP. In practice, there are significant constraints to this freedom (see Chapter 8), but it remains the case that patients register with one individual GP, and it is thus possible to speak of the GP as a personal physician providing care to all who are registered with her or him. An allied notion is that of the family doctor; indeed, general practice is sometimes referred to as 'family medicine'. Both appellations are important as they act as reminders of the close contact with and knowledge of the health needs and problems of an individual patient that a GP may have. Over time, this relationship can have valuable implications for continuity of care and for the appreciation of the social, economic and geographical contexts that constrain patients' health and their responses to treatment.

However, seeing a GP as a personal physician or a family doctor is also deeply problematic. Although the terms may hint at the continuing role of personal advisor in much more than health and illness that many GPs undoubtedly pursue, they are generally outdated. Even though individuals register with one GP, their visits to the surgery are more than likely to result in consultations with any one of the GPs working within the particular GP practice – or even with a person who is not a GP. Furthermore, many of the people who are seen by GPs are not active members of a functioning family unit and, even if they are, the other members of the family may be enrolled with a different GP. As Freeman and Richards (1990) suggest, it may be more accurate to think of practice-based rather than doctor-based continuity of care.

A final general point to be made about UK GPs concerns their status relationship to the NHS. They are, for the most part, independent contractors to the NHS; exceptions to this status are increasing but remain rare (see Chapter 10). Independent contractor status means that GPs sell their services to the NHS on the basis of a nationally agreed contract that is subject to periodic revision. They are not directly employed by the NHS and do not draw fixed salaries. Instead, they share the profits and losses accruing from the operation of their particular practice. Bosanquet and Salisbury (1998) have suggested that this effectively means that they are best seen as owners of small businesses. As such, they face, alongside the demands resulting from patient care, the various pressures consequent upon seeking to run a business dependent on the public sector purse for its income stream. One result of this has been that as the political emphasis has shifted towards general practice so pressures have risen on the business side.

Moving from generalisations to more specific matters, government statistics (OHE 1995) suggest that there were just under 31,000 GPs practising in the UK in the mid-1990s. This figure represents around half of all qualified practising doctors and is roughly double the size of the population of hospital consultants. Within the GP population, nearly 29,000 were practising as what are known as unrestricted GP principals, fully qualified autonomous, 'own-account' practitioners who provide a full range of services to a list that is not restricted to particular types of people. The remainder may work as 'restricted principals', fully qualified in every respect but undertaking limited practice, for example working for an institution or only with a particular type of patient, as Assistants (who may be salaried by the practice rather than partners sharing out profits or losses) or as Trainees.

In terms of age and sex, the GP population at the turn of the millennium has two interesting emerging characteristics. First, in terms of age, nearly 60 per cent of the GP population is aged over 40 (Parkhouse 1991). While this may superficially seem to indicate that general practice is delivered by older people, it must be remembered that GPs tend not to enter practice until their late twenties. Only about one-third of their working life is contained in the period before a fortieth birthday. The implication is therefore that, in reality, GPs are now tending to be younger people – like those other popular pillars of the community, police officers and the clergy. Second, in terms of gender, 31 per cent of GPs are now female (OHE 1997). This figure has risen by 50 per cent over the past decade but masks a continuing lack of equality of opportunity. Parkhouse (1991) shows how 61 per cent of women become principals within 10 years of qualifying while the figure for men is around 90 per cent. The increasing number of women GPs and the relatively lower proportion of women with principal status also underpins a changing work pattern. While male GPs remain predominantly full time, more than 50 per cent of women GPs are working part time.

The major element in any GP's income is a reflection of a capitation fee, a payment for the number of registered patients, around 60 per cent of most incomes being capitation derived. Personal list sizes vary greatly, and in many cases it is more useful to think in terms of practice lists rather than personal lists. In the mid-1990s, the mean list size of an individual unrestricted GP was approximately 1,800 (OHE 1995). Rogers *et al.* (1999) suggest that nearly 80 per cent of the registered population contact a general practice at least once a year. Of those contacting a general practice, most make repeat consultations; the national average per year according to *The General Household Survey* is five (ONS 1995 and annually). The same source also shows that the propensity to consult a GP varies with social class, although the exact nature of this variation is by no means clear. Any analysis of GP consultations by class needs to take account of the class-related nature of the need for GP services. Crudely, lower social status people are more likely to suffer health problems and thus more likely to use a GP. The Black Report (DHSS 1980) addressed this problem by calculating use–need ratios, which indicate that, in general, lower social status people make less use of GP services than they need.

Cartwright and O'Brien (1976) are persistently cited as providers of key evidence concerning the basis for this class-related aspect of GP activity. They note the middle-class background of most GPs and, by implication, suggest that middle-class people and middle-class problems may get more attention and be better understood. Certainly, in a crude empirical sense, it appears from their study that middle-class patients receive consultations that last, on average, a minute and a half longer. Furthermore, middle-class patients tend to ask more of their GPs, and their GPs know more about them. Powell (1997) is sceptical of the robustness of this conclusion but concurs with its general thrust by noting that 'a patient's felt need will lead to no further action if it does not correspond to a GP's concept of normative need' (p. 123). Whatever the extent of class inequality in GP consultation, it is however clear that, overall, there is substantial satisfaction with the service. Cartwright's major studies (Cartwright 1967, Cartwright and Anderson 1981) suggested that over 90 per cent of the population are content with their GP.

What then comprises the average GP workload? There is, of course, no such thing as an average GP, let alone an average workload. What individual GPs do will be dependent on their position within the practice, the length of time since they joined that practice, and their particular interests within the practice, as well as on the location of the practice and a host of other factors. Leaving all these issues aside, valuable general evidence is provided by two sources: Fry's research for the Nuffield Provincial Hospitals Trust (Fry 1991) and the *Fourth National Study of Morbidity in General Practice* (McCormick *et al.* 1995).

Fry was concerned with time use by GPs. Although his figures are now somewhat dated, they are still indicative of what occurs. He found GPs working a 42-hour week of formal activity and a further 23 hours 'on call', during which they could be contacted for work purposes. Deputising services or cooperative arrangements with other practices were increasingly providing cover for the 'on-call' part of this activity. Between 70 and 80 per cent of the workload entailed direct patient contact through surgery- or home-based consultations. The remainder of the GPs' time was spent on practice administration, meetings with external bodies, personal training and the training of others. It was estimated that direct patient contact was some 20 per cent higher in general practice compared with hospital medicine.

McCormick *et al.* (1995) focus on what and whom GPs see during these periods of direct patient contact. Respiratory complaints make up around a third of all consultations. These can range from minor coughs and sneezes through severe influenza and asthma, to life-threatening breathing disorders and lung cancer. Mental health problems are the second most common reason for consulting the GP. Not surprisingly, there is a degree of predictability in the socio-demographic groups most likely to consult. Much of any GP's workload will be dominated by consultations concerning the health problems of people on the practice lists who are either under four or over 75 years of age. Outside these two age groups, the GP is most likely to see women patients, largely as a consequence of needs related to contraception and child-birth. Beyond these dominant client groups, there are also other regularities. People who are widowed or divorced are more likely to consult, as are those who live alone or without other adults but with young children. Higher relative rates of consultation are also evident for people from black and Asian ethnic groups, from people who work in industrial employment and from those not in formal paid work. There is, of course, a substantial confounding and overlap between these various groups, but the key picture is one in which those who might be expected to be most in need of GP services do indeed make the most use of those services.

The residential locations of these groups clearly underpin the inevitable geographies of GP consultation. Consultation rates are higher in the north of England, Scotland and Wales. They are also higher in urban areas and in areas dominated by local authority housing. In each of these cases, if a use–need argument is pursued, these higher consultation rates would be expected. Mortality rates are higher in these areas, and the limited available evidence for spatial variations in morbidity would appear to justify higher relative levels of consultation. In an ideal world, these geographies of consultation would be expected to be reflected in a geography of GP service provision; Chapters 6 and 7 pursue this issue in depth. Here it will suffice to say that particular policies have had to be developed both to reward GPs who practise in more deprived areas, where the propensity to consult is greater, and to induce GPs to practise in areas that are under-doctored. It should also be noted that considerable attention has been focused on the shortcomings of general practice in urban areas and the particular difficulties faced in remote rural areas.

Two final points remain to made about the GP consultation. First, at an average of 8.5 minutes long (Fry and Horder 1994), it is inevitably rather cursory and highly focused. That focus is on individual health care needs and largely on a biomedical response. This reality sits a little uneasily with what has been emerging since the 1960s as the theoretical basis for the GP consultation. The psychosocial perspectives of Balint (1957), which have long been emphasised in GP training and continuing education, are difficult to achieve within a short space of time. Equally difficult in practice is what David Armstrong has termed 'biographical medicine' (Armstrong 1979) – an insight into each individual's health problems across his or her lifespan. Despite these shortcomings, however, the view persists that GPs listen, befriend and explain extraordinarily well.

Second, the locus of the GP consultation has changed significantly in recent years. As will be seen in the next chapter, general practice began as a person-to-person contract. The GP would practise alone. Patients would, if possible, visit him (invariably him) at a surgery held in the GP's home. At least for middle-class patients, the home visit was also common. The 1950s and 60s saw the gradual replacement of 'single-handed' practice by group practice, while health centres were developed largely but by no means exclusively through the 1960s and 70s. By 1995, the modal practice was a six-partner practice, some 25 per cent of practices being of this size. Less than 10 per cent of practice remained 'single-handed'. The increasing scale of the GP enterprise was matched by a concentration of consultations into the setting of the surgery. Fewer than 10 per cent of GP consultations are now held in the patient's home (Bosanquet and Salisbury 1998). This has in turn been enabled by developments in care that have meant that patients are now able to be more mobile through their illnesses as a result of greater flexibility in the deployment of non-medical services.

The mention of non-medical services necessitates a further point concerning the context within which GPs now work. As providers of local community-based medical care, they are key members of a team with responsibilities extending across health and related areas of social care: the primary health care team. What exactly primary care is has been a matter of some debate. Given the nature of the 'clinical iceberg' – the fact that most ill-health is not treated by the medical system at all and is thus known only to the unhealthy person – true primary care is perhaps best thought of as self-care. More realistically, much primary care is provided by family members, usually women (Graham 1984).

For the World Health Organization (WHO 1978), such familial care is very much part of primary health care. It tends, however, to lie outside the definitions used within the UK NHS. In that context, the primary health care 'team' tends to be thought of as comprising services purchased by statutory agencies to facilitate the health care of people in their own homes (Ministry of Health 1963, Hasler *et al.* 1968, NHSE 1994a, Hasler 1996, Hayden 1996). The team will certainly include GPs, district nurses and health visitors. In an extended definition it can be thought of as including housing and social care professionals and perhaps even community pharmacists. In practice and day-to-day parlance, it is, however, usually limited to the first three named professions. GPs have traditionally dominated within the primary health care team, and official guidance has tended to reinforce this dominance despite paying lip-service to multidisciplinarity (NHSE 1994a). This point is reinforced by reflecting upon the finances of primary care: GP salaries are responsible for about one-third of NHS expenditure on primary care, the drugs they prescribe accounting for a further third (Baggott 1994).

Given these various characteristics, can NHS general practice be thought of as being in any way distinctive? The strict answer to this question must be 'yes'. NHS general practice is distinctive in the way it is organised and in the context in which it operates. A key issue is the relationship between specialism and generalism. The UK GP is a generalist who controls access to specialists and can, as such, play a significant role in rationing hospital care (Harrison and Hunter 1994). In France, Germany and the USA, in contrast, it is possible to access specialists directly and these specialists may well have offices outside hospital in 'primary care' settings. The relationship between general practice and public health provides another point of departure. In the UK, these are separate disciplines, despite the urgings of Julian Tudor Hart that effective general practice demands work with patients' communities as well as with individual patients (Tudor Hart 1988). Again in contrast, public health and general practice are well integrated in Nordic and Iberian countries. Some key points of selective comparison can be derived from Horder (1998) (Table 1.1).

From this table it is clear that, at least with regard to Horder's selection of comparisons, the Netherlands and Denmark are the countries where there is someone who closely resembles the UK GP. Neither of these countries, however, has an overall health care system that is the same as the UK NHS. In both, GPs also tend to practise alone or in pairs rather than in the larger group practices that characterise the UK situation. UK GPs also provide significantly shorter consultations. Looking further afield, it is really only in countries with a long history of links with the UK or with a comparable national health service that anything like the UK GP can really be said to exist.

A Chronology of a Recent Reform

The UK NHS has been the subject of substantial reform over the past few years. No area has escaped change, but some have received greater attention than others. Among these has been general practice. This increasing political

Table 1.1   The distinctiveness of NHS general practice

UK characteristic	Comparisons
Personal registration with a GP	Canada, Denmark, Netherlands, Italy, Portugal, Spain
GPs are generalists	France, Denmark, Netherlands
GPs are gatekeepers for secondary care	Denmark, Netherlands
Few GPs work alone	Sweden
Capitation payment	Denmark, Netherlands, Italy

salience was alluded to above. A continuing goal of the reforms has been the development of a primary care-led NHS in which general practice plays a key role. This has, to some extent, challenged the traditional dominance of secondary (hospital) care in the NHS. In seeking to promote health care that builds upwards from general practice and is 'seamless' to the consumer, the balance of emphasis has inevitably shifted somewhat to primary health care. Chapters 3 and 4 will consider this recent history in depth. In order to establish the magnitude of these recent reforms and to provide a basis for subsequent discussion, Table 1.2 sets out a brief chronology of events.

Table 1.2   Recent health care reforms directly affecting general practice

Year	Reform
1987	*Promoting Better Health: The Government's Programme for Improving Primary Health Care* (the primary care White Paper; DHSS 1987)
1988	*Community Care: Agenda for Action* (DHSS 1988, The Griffiths Community Care Report)
1989	*Working for Patients* (DoH 1989a) Introduction of charges for eye tests and dental inspections *Caring for People: Community Care in the Next Decade and Beyond* (DoH 1989b)
1990	1990 GP contract Family Practitioner Committees reconstituted as Family Health Service Authorities (FHSAs) NHS and Community Care Act
1991	Implementation of the NHS internal market and GP fundholding
1993	Implementation of the community care provisions of the NHS and Community Care Act
1995	Health Authorities Act – abolition of regional health authorities; amalgamation of FHSAs and district health authorities (implemented in 1996)
1996	*Primary Care: Delivering the Future* (DoH 1996a) *Choice and Opportunity: Primary Care – the Future* (DoH 1996b)
1997	Primary Care Act General election: New Labour victory New Labour NHS White Papers: *Designed to Care. Renewing the National Health Service in Scotland* (Scottish Office Department of Health 1997); *The New NHS: Modern, Dependable* (England; DoH 1997)
1998	*NHS Wales: Putting Patients First* (Welsh Office 1998b) *Fit for the Future. The Government's Proposals for the Future of the Health and Personal Social Services in Northern Ireland* (Green Paper for Northern Ireland; DHSS (NI) 1998)
1999	Implementation of primary care groups
2000	First primary care trusts

In talking about the introduction of the NHS in 1948, Godber (1975) placed great emphasis on the role played by general practice: 'it was general practice sustained by 37 years of National Health Insurance and gaining substantial additional support from the new system which really carried the National Health Service at its inception' (p. 5). Much the same could be said about successive Conservative and Labour visions of the NHS through the 1980s and 90s. Without unduly anticipating forthcoming discussion, the therapeutic salience of general practice in the day-to-day operation of the NHS was matched by an increasingly central role in the development of the NHS as a party political project. This political centrality chiefly reflected the position of general practice as the level of the NHS with the greatest claim to closeness to the patient. Policies centred on general practice were presented as being responsive to community needs. By building policies such as GP fundholding and primary care groups around general practice, successive governments sought to harness this supposed organic connection between general practice and local communities.

Two points can be made at this juncture about the political salience of general practice over the past few years. First, although it might be suggested that there has been an opportunistic but well-founded recognition and use of the centrality of the GP to care-giving in the NHS, this recognition can also be located in the wider debate about primary care. The dominant position of GPs in the primary health care team has already been noted, as has the persistent focus of general practice on the care of the individual patient rather than on the more population-focused public health of the community in which the patients live and become sick. The broad primary health concerns of the WHO (1978) are only selectively met by general practice. As Marks (1989) notes, GPs would have to become substantially more population orientated in their approach if they were truly to conform to generally understood notions of primary health care as opposed to primary health medicine.

A second point that needs to be made about the political salience of general practice is that it has not been without costs. Comment has been made above on this issue with reference to administration within the contemporary GP workload. Note should, however, also be taken of the difficulties now faced in GP recruitment, both to partnerships and to vocational training schemes. Williams *et al.* (1993) claim that empirical evidence exists showing that GP job satisfaction declined after the implementation of the 1990 contract and, anecdotally, few people researching with GPs will have escaped a realisation that, as a profession, they feel perennially put-upon by bureaucratic demands. Following Elston (1991), Williams and his colleagues suggest the relevance of two theses: proletarianisation and deprofessionalisation. With the first, the 'burden' of regulation through form-filling and managerial oversight is held to have reduced GPs' cherished autonomy as independent contractors. With the second, the movement towards greater patient involvement in care choices and the push to provide more information to patients has created a consumer population who are more knowledgable about GPs' activities and more critical. Together, proletarianisation and deprofessionalisation serve as a reminder that general practice is now rather more strongly controlled than it has been in the past.

This then is NHS general practice. Through its position as 'first-line' primary care and gatekeeper to secondary hospital care, it is a therapeutic cornerstone to the NHS. The consultation in general practice is a key act in health-seeking behaviour. General practice is a service of some scope and magnitude, and has experienced considerable development over the past century, particularly the past decade.

This Book

Despite being central to the NHS, one of the key pillars of the UK welfare state, GPs and general practice, have received surprisingly little extended book-length study in the social sciences. Certain discrete aspects, particularly the 1990-97 GP fundholding initiative (Glennerster *et al.* 1994), have attracted some attention. Outside a few landmark works, however, notably those of Anne Cartwright (Cartwright 1967, Cartwright and Anderson 1981), John Butler (1987) and David Wilkin (Wilkin *et al.* 1987), general practice has tended to be considered within texts on the grand sweep of health policy rather than in its own right. With the exception of Groenwegen *et al.* (1991), comparative analyses of general practice are conspicuously rare. This picture shifts only slightly if attention is expanded to include books that provide a substantial coverage of general practice within an overall focus on primary care (for example Fry 1988, Meads 1996, Rogers *et al.* 1999), magisterial histories of general practice (Honigsbaum 1979, Loudon *et al.* 1998) or the memoirs and thoughts of GPs (Tudor Hart 1988, Widgery 1991).

This book is intended to contribute to the unmet need for an extended social scientific study of general practice in the UK. It specifically concerns general practice and GPs rather than the more general issue of primary care, and reports the authors' own research in the geography of health care and health policy, as well as synthesising the work of others. The intention is to be critical but informative, focusing on the implications of policy developments and the consequences for the future of general practice. The structure of the book falls naturally into three parts: an historical assessment of the development of general practice, an analysis of contemporary themes and a conclusion examining future scenarios and comparative issues.

Chapters 2, 3 and 4 comprise the historical study, the emphasis being on more recent years. Chapter 2 considers the historical origins of general practice and the nature of the 'independent contractor' status. In temporal terms, it covers the period up to the 1987 White Paper. Its historical sweep is thus extensive and includes consideration of the administration of 'executive council services', the development of group practices and the concept of the primary care team, as well as pre-NHS history. Prevention is the theme pursued in Chapter 3. That chapter examines the role of general practice in the prevention of ill-health, focusing particularly on the landmark 1987 White Paper and the 1990 GP contract. Specific attention is given to GP remuneration as driven by the 1990 contract with regard to health promotion, screening activity and childhood immunisation. Chapter 4 is a bridge to more recent issues. It considers the 1990 NHS reforms and subsequent developments in so far as they have impacted upon general practice. Particular attention is given to GP fundholding and to the successor notions of health care commissioning and the primary care group. Central to the chapter will be an analysis of the benefits and shortcomings of a system that has moved GPs to a position of some power with regard to the purchase of secondary care.

Chapters 5–9 are thematic and have been selected to enable a focus on core themes in the delivery of general practice services. Attention is given first to GP accountability. As was noted above, general practice is now more substantially regulated than was once the case. Chapter 5 considers how this is done, contrasting the increased role of patients with managerially led accountability, notions of clinical governance and the role of external bodies such as the Audit Commission. Chapter 6 turns the spotlight on general practice in its community context. It reflects on policies designed to ensure equity in the distribution of GP services and reward for GPs serving deprived areas. This broadly geographical focus is continued in Chapter 7, where a contrast is drawn between urban and rural general practice. The particular problems of working in inner city and remote rural areas are assessed, and policy responses are critically evaluated. GP–patient relationships, consumerism and choice are the themes of Chapter 8. Consideration is given to the extent to which patient choice really exists within general practice. We examine increased expectations of and demands on GPs, as well as complaints systems and 'problem' patients. The last thematic chapter focuses on GPs and social care. It evaluates GPs' activity in the field of community care management and assesses the effectiveness of their interface with social services departments.

The book concludes with a single chapter concentrating on the prognosis for UK general practice. We look at innovations in the UK context that challenge traditional perspectives of what general practice is about and also briefly examine the parallels, problems and lessons that can be learned from overseas, particularly from the Netherlands, the nearest European parallel to the UK general practice system, from New Zealand, where so much of New Labour policy has originated, and from the USA.

2

The Development of General Practice – from Potions to Purchasing

In the current NHS, the role of primary care, and in particular that of the GP, is seen as pivotal. The bulk of patient care is provided by the GP or members of the primary health care team, such as the practice nurse, health visitor or district nurse. With the exception of those patients who are admitted to hospital from accident and emergency departments, all individuals requiring hospital treatment must be referred by a GP. In addition, since the NHS reforms in 1990, GPs' views on the effectiveness of hospital and community services have carried considerable weight in the management of local services. Yet the current status that general practice enjoys as a speciality within medicine and the influence that GPs wield are in sharp contrast with its origins and much of its history, during which general practice was overshadowed by the more prestigious branches of medicine.

This chapter will chart the development of general practice, from its humble origins as a quasi-trade, to the beginnings of its key role in today's health service. In doing so, three interlinking themes will receive particular attention: tensions within the profession – demarcatory conflicts and the 'campaign' for identity; attempts to improve GPs' income and conditions; and the place of general practice in a socialised health care system, together with the consequent dynamics between state and profession. Cule (1980) suggests that the history of general practice extends over a period of 2,000 years. This chapter will confine itself to a more manageable tranche of time. It will explore the period from the early nineteenth century to the creation of the NHS, before focusing on more recent developments, ending with the White Paper *Promoting Better Health* (DHSS 1987). More recent policy initiatives, such as the NHS and Community Care Act and the GP contract, both introduced in 1990, will be explored elsewhere in the book.

Early Beginnings

The profession of medicine evolved from three distinct occupational groups. At the beginning of the nineteenth century, physicians, surgeons and apothecaries each had a governing body: the Royal College of Physicians (RCP), the Royal College of Surgeons (RCS) and the Worshipful Company of Apothecaries. These ordained the type of education or apprenticeship undertaken by entrants, their functions being separately defined in law (Parry and Parry 1976). The system both reflected and institutionalised differences in status between the three types of practitioner. Apothecaries had to surrender membership of the Apothecaries Hall before becoming licensed surgeons, and the RCP required both surgeons and apothecaries to renounce membership of their respective bodies before they could be accepted as licentiates of the RCP. The differing status of physicians, surgeons and apothecaries influenced the nature of their practice and the financial rewards that this yielded. Physicians, who were relatively few in number, were concentrated in London and the larger provincial towns, and had lucrative practices among the rich. Those, however, who were licentiates rather than fellows of the Royal College were forced to adopt a more generalist approach to practice. Surgeons also served the wealthy, but in the days before anaesthesia and antisepsis, surgery was considered a last resort rather than being offered as a treatment of choice. By 1829, the apothecary, originally a mere dispenser of dubious medicines, was authorised to charge for medical advice and thus bridged the gap between tradesperson and professional. Honigsbaum (1979) suggests that patients continued to assume that medication would be dispensed following consultation, an expectation that practitioners would maintain still persists. As medical practitioners, apothecaries served the general needs of the middle and lower classes, as well as dispensing medicines for the rich on the prescription of physicians.

Medical training began in the newly established voluntary hospitals that had developed in most major cities during the eighteenth century. These, in addition to the older charitable hospitals, provided for the poor. Physicians and surgeons donated their services for the privilege of honing their doubtful skills on the unsuspecting and unfortunate. It was a system that excluded the humbler apothecary and, with the advancement of medical science, widened the professional division between an increasingly specialist consultant and the predominantly generalist practitioner. These differences enhanced what were, according to Stevens (1966), class divisions, the hierarchy of physicians, surgeons and apothecaries and their practice loci becoming well established by 1800. Hospital practice became the setting for research and teaching, and access to beds the currency of prestige and power. It preceded and survived the movement to coordinate the profession's regulation of training and qualification, and was reinforced by the further gradual exclusion of GPs from local hospitals in the inter-war years (see below).

The formal divisions between apothecaries and surgeons were the first to weaken as surgical techniques developed (Honigsbaum 1979) and as the urbanisation of society and population growth created a growing demand for medical care, provided by the 'prototype general practitioners' (Cherry 1996:27). In 1815, the Apothecaries Act formalised the apprenticeship of apothecaries and established rudimentary examinations for qualification, successful candidates becoming licentiates of the Society of Apothecaries. Despite not being required to obtain dual qualifications, namely membership of the RCS and the Licence of the Society of Apothecaries (LSA), 95 per cent of newly qualified doctors did so (Cherry 1996). In the 1830s, the movement to promote a unified, self-regulated profession out of the disorder created by competition between the traditional organising bodies gained momentum and was particularly popular among the rising number of GPs, who sought the same status in society as the fellows of the RCP (Parry and Parry 1976). The aspiring profession was also plagued by competition from other occupations, such as pharmacists, and by a number of unqualified hacks. The latter were regarded as a threat to the medical practitioner's credibility, although the legitimacy of this claim is difficult to sustain since most medical treatments at this time were of doubtful efficacy.

Common professional status and professional self-regulation were eventually achieved in the Medical Registration Act of 1858 after protracted and tortuous negotiations between the three practitioner groups. At issue were the educational requirements of practitioners and the jurisdiction of the organising bodies. Various options were proposed, including one that would have required all members of the profession to qualify as GPs before they could qualify as specialists. These and other suggestions were abandoned in the face of opposition from one or other of the three bodies, who were determined to defend the interests of their members. The eventual Bill resulted in a single register of practitioners, but the Royal Colleges and the Apothecaries Hall continued as a separate means of entry to the profession. A General Council of Medical Education and Registration was created to establish standards of education and determine entry to the register. As Parry and Parry (1976) suggest, the equal recognition before the law of those qualifying from the three organising bodies provided the basis for unification. This levelling effect appealed to many entrants to the profession but disconcerted the élite, well-established and well-heeled physicians, and did nothing to resolve continuing tensions between the three groups of practitioner. Nor did the separate qualifications guarantee competency for general practice. According to Cule (1980), the LSA and the membership examinations of the RCS were each deficient in specific areas of practice. This was accommodated if the practitioner elected to take both qualifications, but the requirement to take a conjoint diploma was not introduced until 1884. As such, it became the recognised qualification for GPs during the next 50 years.

The 1858 Medical Registration Act was an exclusory measure designed to protect the market interests of the profession, which in turn operated internal demarcations between specialist consultants and lower-status generalists. The Act, however, also has to be seen in terms of the nineteenth-century state's attempt to order an increasingly complex and rapidly changing society. Given the prevailing liberalist values, which fiercely proscribed the state's incursion into commerce, self-regulation of the profession was the only conceivable option. It is a position that governments have continued to support, although the central and local state's involvement in public health measures and in the provision of health care, initially to the indigent and since 1948 to the whole population, has clearly been influential in determining the organisation of medical work.

State Provision and the General Practitioner

The public health reforms provide one piece of evidence about the changing conceptualisation of the state and the individual. The increasing involvement in public health provision reflected philanthropic concerns about the waves of epidemics that ravaged the populations of the new industrial towns, but this was matched by the rather mercantilist perception that disease was weakening the labour force. A number of public health acts from 1848 onwards meant that, by the 1875 Public Health Act, minimum sanitary requirements had been established. The responsibility for attaining these was charged to local authorities. From 1872, Medical Officers of Health (MOHs) were to be appointed in each authority. A central authority, the Local Government Board, was responsible for the overall administration of public health measures and combined these duties with the supervision of the Poor Law, taking over the responsibilities of the former Poor Law Board. It executed the latter with little enthusiasm (Brand 1965).

After the 1858 Medical Registration Act, 'Outdoor' relief for the poor could be provided only by qualified doctors, who usually combined it with other forms of contractual practice in order to make a living. There was competition for posts in some parts of the country, a state of affairs frequently exploited by the local Boards of Guardians to control costs; the Poor Law doctor was often expected to supply medication out of his salary. Nor did he have much professional autonomy, the entitlement of the recipient to Poor Law medical care being regularly at the discretion of the local Board. Because of the inattention of the Local Government Board to these matters, Boards of Guardians, which were inclined to adopt an extremist interpretation of the principle of less eligibility, exercised considerable power. Friction between them and the medical officer was not infrequent (Brand 1965, Parry and Parry 1976). Dissatisfaction with the fortune of the medical officer, the standard of medical care and the tyranny of the local Boards of Guardians was to continue, generating a collective memory that fuelled the desire for autonomy in years to come. Thus, the GP's lot contrasted starkly with that of consultant physicians and surgeons in the voluntary hospitals, who wielded much power at ward and committee level.

The Poor Law regime was attenuated, but not eradicated, by the 1911 National Insurance Act, which marked an advance in the state's involvement in personal, as opposed to public, health services. It provided access to adequate health care for the working population, some of whom would otherwise have required Poor Law support, but, in the eyes of many GPs, this replaced one form of bureaucratic oppression with another.

Outdoor Poor Law work was not the primary source of income for most GPs. Their preference was for private, family doctoring (Cherry 1996). A relatively small number of GPs worked in the more lucrative areas of London and provincial towns, often in competition with specialist physicians. Those doctors whose patients could not afford to pay on each occasion for services rendered often established clubs whereby patients made regular weekly contributions. Commonplace by the 1850s, however, were the clubs run by friendly societies, mutual aid societies and employers. Medical coverage was offered by all three types, but the friendly societies also offered sickness or injury benefits and help with funeral expenses. Competition for posts was fierce and often tainted by corruption. Not infrequently, auctions for medical officer posts ensured that the position went to the lowest bidder, who was then often prepared to provide only minimal care. This gave rise to concern and the prevailing opinion, noted by Sidney and Beatrice Webb in 1910, that the club doctor was an inferior type of practitioner (Brand 1965). For their part, doctors chafed at the nature of their relationships with the friendly societies and club organisations, which cast doctors in the role of hired hands rather than professional practitioners. The societies and clubs exploited the medical labour market and, GPs argued, further reduced doctors' income by diverting some better-off patients who could afford to pay privately. Together with the experiences of the system of Outdoor relief, work as a contract doctor poisoned the GP's view of both the state and the independent organisation as a potential employer. This aversion was to characterise negotiations in future state enterprises in health care provision.

1911–48: Quiescence and Conflict

The National Insurance Act of 1911 and the creation of the NHS in 1948 provide the boundaries of a period which, for the speciality of general practice, was marked by an erosion of clinical practice and a concomitant decline in prestige. This process was not catalysed by state-directed changes in the organisation of medical practice, but was the result of pressure from the consultants in hospital-based specialities who were concerned at the apparent inability or unwillingness of GPs to keep up with developments in clinical practice (Honigsbaum 1979). State initiatives, however, did impact on the work of GPs. The 1911 National Insurance Act was designed to insure the family breadwinner against the disastrous effects of illness and to return him or her to work as quickly as possible – thereby ending the state's provision of financial support. Contributions entitled participants to register with a GP selected from a panel for medical advice and treatment but excluded coverage for most hospital care. The state's first significant foray into health care did not, therefore, encroach on the territory of the hospital-based consultant.

GPs, however, feared the effects of state provision on the market for private medicine. They were irritated by the government's lack of consultation and appalled by its intention to administer the scheme through approved friendly societies and work-related insurance companies, which seemed to be a regeneration of previous arrangements (Brand 1965, Cule 1980, Cherry 1996). Opposition was vehement and sustained, particularly over the issue of remuneration, and persisted until well after the passing of the Act. Despite this, GPs lacked the political sophistication and cohesion that was to characterise the profession in the latter half of the century and were largely excluded from the policy-making agenda. There were, however, distinct benefits to the new arrangements, and the resistance of the profession's leaders was undermined by a slow trickle of GPs won over to the new scheme by the prospect of improved earnings. GPs were given representation on the administrative committees and permitted autonomy of clinical practice, something they had not enjoyed in Poor Law or club practice. They were paid a capitation fee, separate from treatment costs, producing a significant increase in income (Livingstone and Widgery 1990). Moreover, competition for patients, which had previously existed between the GP and hospital specialists and which had only been tempered by the practice of referral,[1] abated.

Honigsbaum characterised the period as one in which the potential for further innovation and improvement in general practice was lost because of the profession's indifference. The Dawson Report, published in 1920, conceived doctors as working in group practices, offering extensive and up-to-date services. The proposal initially won the partial support of the British Medical Association (BMA), which saw in it a means of relieving a major source of GP grievance: the 24-hour contractual obligation under the National Health Insurance (NHI) scheme and night calls in particular. This is a complaint that still persists today. Despite the BMA's view that health centres might be beneficial for deprived areas, where practice conditions were woefully inadequate, it was opposed to their universal application. As

Dawson developed his original concept into something altogether more elaborate, the opposition of GPs grew. They objected to the proposal to include inpatient (GP) beds without additional pay. In particular, they feared the spectre of a salaried service and the involvement of local authorities in the person of the MOHs, who were to be located in health centres (Honigsbaum 1979). Several decades later, support for the concept of group practices was revived as part of a more general movement to improve conditions in and the stature of general practice.

Although GPs had long been excluded from the larger hospitals, they retained clinical control in the rural cottage hospitals, where they could practise both medicine and surgery. The opportunity to consolidate GP clinical practice within the hospitals was presented when, in 1929, the Local Government Act abolished the Boards of Guardians and placed the Poor Law infirmaries under the control of local authority MOHs. In addition, many local authorities, perhaps galvanised by these new responsibilities, exercised powers granted under the 1875 Public Health Act and built general hospitals. As a consequence, they had by the end of the 1930s emerged as major hospital administrations (Webster 1988).

Instead of allowing GPs access to the municipal hospitals, since the MOHs' experiences of GP cooperation and performance in local authority hospitals were mainly poor, many MOHs chose to staff them with specialist physicians and surgeons from the voluntary sector hospitals. Those provincial authorities which were forced to use GPs because of a shortage of specialists 'often had cause for regret' (Honigsbaum 1979:139). Worse still, responsibility for the high maternal mortality rates of the inter-war period was placed at the door of GPs. Hospital consultants, particularly surgeons, were reluctant to permit GP hospital practice. In the words of one former hospital doctor, 'GPs were regarded almost as members of another profession, and pretty inferior ones at that' (Gibson 1981:51). GPs had done little to improve the situation by rejecting the principle of assessment for hospital specialist competence in 1928 (Honigsbaum 1979).

The development of private insurance schemes for hospital care from the 1920s onwards, which tended to specify consultant care, further excluded GPs from hospital practice, although they retained more than a professional toe-hold in paediatrics and anaesthetics, the Conjoint Board offering diplomas in each from 1935. The resulting ill-feeling caused by the reluctant exodus of some GPs from hospital-based medicine rejuvenated old divisions within the profession; general practice had reached its nadir.

Alternative careers had to be found. By the early 1940s, consultants were encouraging the idea of group general practices that would focus on preventive and public health, leaving curative medicine in the hands of hospital specialists. In addition, paediatricians, who were dissatisfied with the performance of local authority clinics, urged GPs to concentrate on child welfare.

This initially caused concern among obstetric specialists, who had been highly critical of GPs' maternity care, but they did not object to an involvement after the infant had survived to 10 days (Honigsbaum 1979), a proposal that carries the faint suggestion that GPs were to be restrained until the child had a sporting chance of survival. GPs gradually abandoned the idea of a specialist clinical role rooted in general practice but, by accepting their role as generalists catering for less exotic conditions, yielded a great service to the future NHS. In noting the relative absence of generalists within the US medical profession, Stevens (1966) concludes that the absence of the referral system and the resulting competition provided every incentive to specialise. In contrast, the division of labour that allocated a separate function to the GP – that of provider of mainstream medical services and gatekeeper to secondary care – ensured the viability of general practice.

Despite being left with little to specialise in other than general practice, there was scant interest in innovation. Support for a new initiative in group practice was lukewarm, with 'Most doctors [seeming] to work on the unjustifiable assumption that isolated practice [was] somehow intrinsic to medicine' (Eckstein 1958:80). A more accurate assessment might be that group practice was perceived to be intrinsically linked to local authority administration. However, other events disrupted deliberations in the 1940s. During World War Two, expectations of the state's role in welfare changed and plans for a state health service began to crystallise.

The idea of a national health service had been proposed – and quashed – in Parliament as early as 1834 and had subsequently been periodically aired (Brand 1965, Cule 1980). After World War One, political attention became increasingly focused on the issue as the financial condition of the voluntary hospitals became more pressing and pressure grew for a comprehensive public service. As planning for World War Two got under way, the disorganised state of medical services was very evident. Some problems proved insurmountable and persisted throughout the war. However, the experience of many doctors involved in the Emergency Medical Service changed their impression of working within a state-run service (Titmuss 1963). A consensus for a state-provided health service had been developing since the 1920s, but the climate of opinion following the Allied victory was such that some form of national health service was considered the inalienable right of the British people. More extensive accounts of the tortuous negotiations and various blueprints generated can be found in Webster (1988), Eckstein (1958), Willcocks (1967) and Klein (1995), for example.

The concern here is with the involvement of the GPs' lobby, which, along with the voluntary hospitals' lobby, reacted strongly to the tentative suggestion of a salaried service early in discussions. The campaign was spearheaded by the BMA, which still brooded on its defeat over NHI and subsequent skirmishes with government, and was implacably opposed to anything smacking of state control (Webster 1988). Negotiations therefore proceeded on the premise of government maleficence towards the profession. No doubt the GPs' experience with the administration of NHI coloured their view of local bureaucracies; their abiding fear was of being placed under the (salaried) control of local authorities, which they caricatured as parochial and stultifying.

Aneurin Bevan, the Minister of Health charged with creating the NHS in post-war Britain, entered into separate and successful negotiations with the consultants. They refused to be represented by the BMA, reopening the historical rift between themselves and GPs, who were thus isolated. The consultants gained from negotiations, achieving independent status for the teaching hospitals and a recognition of their pivotal role in the governance of the NHS. Forsyth (1966) argues that the relationship between consultants and GPs changed significantly after 1948 as consultants were no longer reliant on the referral of patients by GPs for their income, a lever that was to some extent to reappear in the GP fundholding scheme introduced in 1990.

Bevan made some concessions to the sensitivities of GPs over professional independence and proposed local executive committees, with whom GPs would contract their services, and a remuneration scheme based on a combination of capitation fees and salary. Two other proposals, that GPs should no longer buy and sell their practices and that a central committee should have the power to prevent doctors establishing practices in over-doctored areas, were seen as being less conciliatory. The BMA reacted strongly and mustered sufficient support among GPs to threaten the start of the NHS, planned for July 1948. In the event, the Presidents of the Royal Colleges of Surgeons and Physicians persuaded the BMA to adopt a more conciliatory approach, and opposition to the NHS ceased (Eckstein 1958).

Whether the footsoldiers understood the tactics of the whole campaign is difficult to ascertain. Gibson perhaps speaks for many when he describes his feelings at the time. He describes:

> being just a pawn in a rather bewildering game, in which the rules were partly dictated and partly made up from week to week. I doubt if any of us in general practice then fully realised how our discipline was to be isolated and denigrated. (1981:71)

The NHS settlement allowed GPs to retain their status as independent contractors, although the autonomy that this implies was blunted by the reality that the state operated a virtual monopsony, private general practice having all but disappeared as the result of the nationalised service. Mass resignation from the service threatened the introduction of the NHS and was used as industrial leverage in subsequent negotiations over pay and conditions, but in practical terms it threatened disruption, from which many doctors shrank, rather than a genuine option of exit. Moreover, the new arrangements carried some benefits: many GPs were relieved to be rid of the task of collecting debts from non-panel patients, a practice that served in lieu of an adequate pension in retirement (Raistrick 1988), and the system appeared to offer greater financial security than before.

All was not well, however. General practice at the beginning of the NHS was isolated both professionally and in administrative terms because Executive Councils were separate from the Regional Hospital Boards and local Hospital Management Committees, reflecting the traditional separation of voluntary hospitals from local authority and National Insurance-based health care. GPs largely practised in single-handed or two-doctor practices and had little contact with the teaching hospitals. Without such contact, it proved difficult to maintain an acceptable level of knowledge in a rapidly developing science. Practice premises had to be purchased and maintained at the personal expense of the GP, as had the salaries of any ancillary staff employed. As in other parts of the service, general practice was overwhelmed by a flood of previously unmet demands for health care and standards fell (Gibson 1988).

The publication of research highly critical of general practice (Collings, cited in Stevens 1966, Webster 1988) produced a strong reaction. Collings, noting the marginalisation of general practice from the remainder of medicine, stated that the quality of practice was unsatisfactory and deteriorating. The survey sample could be faulted but 'most of his shots hit their mark with explosive impact' (Webster 1988:356). Two further studies produced contradictory findings, but research by Taylor (cited in Petchey 1995) of 'best' practices concluded that about 25 per cent of those were unsatisfactory. Thus, the long-held perception of the wider profession, that the descendants of the nineteenth-century apothecary were inferior members, appeared to have been vindicated.

The New Practitioner

The creation of the College of General Practitioners in 1952 began to encourage an academic coherence in the discipline and, according to Hasler (1992), promoted primary health care teams as well as other improvements. Despite this, the morale of the profession continued to deteriorate in the 1950s and early 1960s. The source of much discontent was the terms of the contract, which set out the pay and conditions for general practice. A complicated 'pool' system had operated since 1948, the total amount of which was calculated on a notional average net income per GP. The formula included a sum for practice expenses (the amount being taxable), but other income (for example, private income and that from clinical assistantships in hospitals), which *some* GPs received, was subtracted from the total pool to be dispersed among all practising GPs. The total net income was also calculated on the number of GPs in the pool rather than of the population. As Forsyth (1966) observes, the system operated on the concept of an average GP with an average number of patients and an average range of additional work. Those doctors who relied to a greater extent on capitation payments for income got a raw deal, and subsequent pay awards were converted to a smaller rise in income once the award had been processed through the pool formula. Because it did not directly reimburse practice expenditure, the system discouraged an improvement to premises and an outlay on staff support.

Dissatisfaction grew with these arrangements and with the growing gulf between specialists' incomes and those of GPs (Forsyth 1966), and was not ameliorated by successive pay awards made by the Review Body in 1963 and 1964. Fraught and protracted negotiations between the profession's representative bodies, the government and the Review Body continued. In 1965, the BMA's Annual Representative Meeting approved the Family Doctors' Charter, which demanded, among other things, the abolition of the pool and the 24-hour obligatory service, support for the purchase or improvement of practice premises, reimbursement in full of the costs of ancillary staff, and fees for service in relation to weekend and night visits.

Kenneth Robinson, the then Minister of Health, attempted in negotiations to accentuate the benefits of introducing group practices with attached local authority nurses, midwives and health visitors, measures not related to remuneration (Webster 1996). The GPs were not to be deflected, and Robinson, largely sympathetic to their claims, agreed to negotiate on the basis of the Charter. The first measure to be introduced, in October 1965, was the direct reimbursement of practice staff. Other gains followed: reimbursement of the costs of practice rents; financial inducements to work in under-doctored areas; and additional payments, such as the basic practice allowance and seniority payments, the latter conditional on the GP undertaking periodic refresher courses. There was to be a range of payments for items of service, and three categories of capitation fee related to age were to reflect the assumed different demands of patients for the GP's time. Night and weekend services also attracted an additional payment, but the government refused to accept responsibility for organising these. These contractual arrangements persisted with only minor modification until the 'new' GP contract was imposed on a hostile profession by the Conservative government in 1990 .

The introduction of substantive elements of the Family Doctors' Charter has been hailed as a turning point in the resourcing of general practice (Livingstone and Widgery 1990) and in the recognition and encouragement of good practice (Gibson 1988). However, the search for a professional identity and role continued. According to Honigsbaum (1979), specialists, determined to keep GPs out of hospital medicine, emphasised the requirement to coordinate health care in the community. There was a growing need to provide care for the chronic sick, whose numbers were swelled by an ageing population. In addition, advances in therapeutics meant that some patients with long-term illness could be maintained outside long-stay institutions, which had been tainted by a Poor Law ancestry. As early as 1957, GPs had been identified in a Ministry of Health report as being key elements in the development of community care (Boucher, cited in Honigsbaum 1979).

Group practice was becoming the norm (Livingstone and Widgery 1990), and from the 1950s onwards some forward-looking MOHs introduced the 'attachment' of local authority nurses (district nurses, health visitors and midwives) to practices (Hasler 1992). Gibson (1981) describes how, in negotiations over the Family Doctor's Charter, Kenneth Robinson sought to encourage the model of a group practice with attached staff. This initiative was enjoying limited success in some parts of the country: Hampshire had 160 family doctors with workers attached. The concept of attached staff was, however, not always warmly received. A 1964 survey by the Wessex Regional Hospital Board found that fewer than 50 per cent of GPs wanted health visitors attached (Hasler 1992), although this may have reflected the profession's view of the health visitor's worth (and possibly that of preventive medicine) rather than being a rejection of the attachment of nursing staff *per se*.

Urged on by the profession's leaders as well as the government, more and more GPs participated in local authority attachment schemes. The larger premises made affordable by the cost rents scheme facilitated the attachment of staff, and the 70 per cent reimbursement allowance encouraged the employment of administrative support staff and practice nurses (Stilwell 1991, Hasler 1992). Further encouragement for the development of attached teams came with the 1974 reorganisation of the health service. This resulted in local authorities losing their responsibilities for health care, with the exception of environmental health services. Nursing staff were transferred to community nursing departments, and subsequently located in practices, rather than being deployed along the lines of the previous arrangement of geographical coverage within the local authority. Practice attachment was meant to facilitate a team approach to delivering family health care – as opposed to general practice medicine. Attached nursing staff, and the later growth of practice-employed nurses, thus made feasible the development of, at its best, a needs-led, comprehensive and efficient primary care system offering more than the sum of its professional parts. However, the underpinning concept of the primary health care team was, for many community nurses, insufficiently realised. The conditions considered necessary for effective primary health care teams, and outlined in the Harding Report (DHSS 1981a), were often found lacking. The Cumberlege Report (DHSS 1986a), which trawled nursing opinion, reflected a disenchantment with the *status quo* in proposing the withdrawal of the 70 per cent reimbursement of practice nurse salaries and a return to geographical 'patch' nursing teams. This, predictably, met with stiff opposition from GPs, among whom there was a high degree of support for staff attachment, if not a complete understanding of the meaning of teamworking. To the disappointment of many community nurses, the Cumberlege Report was rejected.

Burgeoning Speciality, Growing Government Interest

According to Pereira Gray (1994), the problems facing general practice in the late 1960s were the attainment of a research base for the growing academic discipline and the creation of an appropriate post-registration training for GPs. Both were realised over the next decade and a half. There was a need to define the core of general practice and to differentiate it from other forms. Balint (1964) began to construct a theory of clinical general practice, the focus of which was the consultation but which extended to broader family dynamics. Further advances were made with the introduction in 1982 of a mandatory three-year training for those wishing to enter general practice. In addition, departments of general practice became integral elements of most faculties of medicine by the mid-1980s (Pereira Gray 1994).

Interest in a wider interpretation of general practice to include traditional public health concerns of population-based medicine was prompted by the Black Report (DHSS 1980) and the work of Tudor Hart among others. Rudimentary information technology was first introduced into general practice in the early 1970s, but its real potential – the ability to systematise and interrogate richly detailed practice-based information – only began to be exploited in the 1980s in pioneering practices. Tudor Hart's *A New Kind of Doctor* (1988) described a model of proactive general practice that harnessed information technology to identify and screen at-risk groups of patients. Thus, in many ways, the 1980s saw the fruition of many interlinking developments in general practice on which the government was later to capitalise in its drive to establish a primary care-led NHS. It was maturing into a distinct and self-confident speciality, the provision of which was increasingly located in purpose-built premises. The exception to this was inner city general practice, where inadequate conditions obtained and where, according to Marks (1987:1) 'the lowest standards coexist(ed) with the greatest needs'.

The medical profession was regarded by government as a formidable opponent in negotiations, as some of the events described in this chapter demonstrate. In the 1980s, Conservative governments had the recent reminder of the battle over pay beds between Barbara Castle, the then Secretary of State for Social Services, and the consultants. In the end, Castle was forced to back down by the then Prime Minister, Harold Wilson, who was unwilling to persist in the increasingly bitter confrontation. Limiting private practice within the confines of NHS property was patently not one of the missions of the Conservative government, but controlling the expenditure of the welfare state and improving the performance of its constituent parts most certainly was. The NHS, with an approximate expenditure of £7.25m in 1978/79 was a prime target, but while the resourcing of hospital and community services could be subjected to restraints, the open-ended nature of the Family Practitioner Services (FPSs) was another matter. Expenditure in these areas was increasing at a rate faster than that of the remainder of the NHS and, in order to control the increase, it was necessary for the government to trespass on sacred ground: clinical practice. The publication of a limited list of medicines in 1984 constituted a milder form of political assault on GP autonomy, given that it was not possible to impose cash limits on prescribing. Even so, the attempts to weed out ineffective prescribing and also to encourage the substitution of expensive, branded medicines by cheaper, generic alternatives met with predictable opposition from both the profession and the pharmacological industry.

Unabashed by the angry reaction of the profession, the government turned its attention to the management of general practice within the NHS. The changes recommended by Griffiths (DHSS 1983) in the hospital and community health services sector were well underway, and the Conservative government was keen to improve the performance of the FPSs. The recommendations in the Green Paper *Primary Health Care: An Agenda for Discussion* (DHSS 1986b), despite being critically received by the profession, were broadly carried forward in the ensuing White Paper, *Promoting Better Health* (DHSS 1987). Its proposals signalled an enhanced framework of administrative accountability (as in the case of targets linked to financial inducements, for vaccination and screening), the mild discipline of consumerism (the simplification of the process of changing GP and the increase of the capitation element of GP income) and stark behaviour modification (financial incentives to undertake child health surveillance and comprehensive elderly care, and to practise in deprived areas, and a requirement to undertake regular postgraduate training).

The White Paper also proposed a new and tougher role for Family Practitioner Committees (FPCs), whose administrators had hitherto been regarded, in Klein's memorable words, as 'managerial eunuchs whose chief responsibilities were to shuffle paper, to pay out money and to keep GPs happy' (1995:166). FPCs were to be more active in monitoring the performance of GPs and in the allocation of resources for practice staff and premises. They were to encourage cost-effective prescribing in general practice, and in their steerage of FPSs they were to take account of public attitudes. The profession had been forewarned of these moves by the content of the earlier Green

Paper, and the BMA 'reacted tetchily' (Klein 1995:166). It was critical of the strengthened managerial role of FPCs, which, it feared, presaged an end to the traditional independence of the profession. The die was, however, cast; the FPCs took up their new responsibilities, and the 1990 GP contract introduced radical changes to the formula of GP payment (see Chapter 3). Although GPs retained a large measure of independence, the state had intervened irrevocably in the day-to-day performance of general practice.

This chapter has charted the often uneven progress of general practice in its attempts to gain credibility and maintain the income of members of the profession. As apothecaries, the original incarnations of GPs were consigned a lowly role and excluded from high-status work in the voluntary hospitals. While medicine as a whole demanded professional autonomy and the economic privileges that accompanied monopoly provision, many GPs were forced to contract for work with Boards of Guardians, sickness societies and, after 1911, NHI Approved Societies. Few could exercise the autonomy that came with a sole concentration on private practice. However, the schism within the profession, which might well have been generated as a result of the demarcation between hospital specialist and GP, did not occur. Neither did the later drift towards specialisation in medicine absorb general practice, as it did in the US. Instead, the system of referral of patients from GP to hospital specialist *for an opinion* provided for functional co-existence and, by default, created a system envied for its relative efficiency and economy.

More recently, general practice has attempted to assert its identity as a speciality having a recognisable professional territory and supported by a coherent body of theory. Despite some progress, it has been persistently viewed as having the lowest status of all the branches of the profession, and its influence over the dispersal of resources in the NHS went, for many years, unnoticed. Although it was the front line of state-organised health care, general practice attracted little attention from governments. This can no doubt be ascribed to the association of medicine with curative, high-technology provision that has traditionally been the domain of the hospital sector and the consultant. The low status and relative 'anonymity' of general practice was converted into limited professional power, but the profession was also victim to its own lack of cohesiveness and conservatism, which at times rendered it unwieldy and unresponsive. There always remained the capacity to withdraw labour, a tactic that was deployed at the inception of the NHS and which has been periodically threatened since, but the use of this reactive and negative mechanism indicated the peripheral position of GPs in the policy-making process.

In the current global search for greater efficiency in the delivery of health care, the potential of primary care to deliver health gains at less cost has been recognised. Primary care in the UK is fortunate in having an extensive and well-developed system of GPs, which for the Conservative governments of the 1980s represented an undermanaged and potentially wasteful resource. More importantly for the profession, GPs later came to be seen as the catalysts for change throughout the NHS. The Conservatives' health care policies marked a watershed for the NHS and especially for general practice, whose influence looks set to continue despite a change of government (see DoH 1997). The remainder of this book explores the policy objectives of the Conservative and Labour governments for health care and, in particular, general practice. It examines the impact of policies on general practice and the populations served, the wider NHS and GPs themselves.

Notes

1. This was an arrangement whereby the GP referred patients for a second opinion and/or more specialist treatment in a hospital setting. Both GP and consultant derived income from this division of labour.

3

Promoting Better Health

Although discussions of the Conservative party's reforms of the NHS usually make much of the 1989 Prime Ministerial Review and the subsequent publication of the White Paper *Working for Patients* (DoH 1989a), as well as the enactment of the NHS and Community Care Act 1990, the reform process actually began far earlier. Two events were particularly significant here. The first was the imposition of general management in 1984–85 following an Independent Inquiry into NHS Management chaired by Roy Griffiths (DHSS 1983). This development, thought by Timmins (1995) to be rather more significant than later reforms, challenged what was, not altogether accurately, seen as the consensual management style prevalent in the NHS of the early 1980s. The replacement of consensus management by general management achieved two things: the introduction of a significant counterweight to medical power within the NHS, and the basis for a growing private sector-influenced culture of performance measurement and competition. While the interaction of general management with the world of general practice was to become increasingly significant as the NHS reform process unfolded during the 1990s, the new culture of performance and competition also had a more immediate impact, providing a basis for the second event, which standard accounts often neglect in their discussions of the NHS reforms. This event was the publication, in 1987, of a White Paper on primary care: *Promoting Better Health* (DHSS 1987).

Promoting Better Health set out some far-reaching changes to the ways in GPs were to work; the previous chapter introduced its key concerns. Most importantly, it underpinned a major reform to the GPs' collective contract with the NHS. The purpose of this chapter is to assess and analyse the proposals set out in *Promoting Better Health* and to reflect upon their precursors, context and consequences. It is essentially a bridge between the more distant historical review set out in Chapter 1 and the analysis of the contemporary policy position of GPs as commissioners that forms the subject matter of Chapter 4. The chapter takes as its central theme the role of GPs in the promotion of health and the prevention of disease. The structure of the chapter is straightforward. The next section examines the White Paper, commencing with an assessment of background factors. Consideration is given to the political environment of the time and the developments that underpinned the primary care proposals. Attention then turns to the actual content of the White Paper and to the extent to which its measures were implemented, most notably in the 1990 GP contract. Debates over this contract are also examined. A set of three case studies are then presented, examining health promotion within the context of the contract: on health promotion clinics, health check screening and immunisation target payments. The chapter concludes with a brief reflection on the state of general practice at the end of the 1980s on the eve of the period more traditionally associated with the reform of the NHS.

The 1987 'Primary Care' White Paper

In much the same way as the NHS reform that commenced in 1989/90 cannot be seen as a sudden unheralded event, the 1987 primary care White Paper did not arise without its own contextual developments and precursors. At least three such background factors can be identified. All were, to a greater or lesser extent, themselves located in the broad and sometimes contradictory framework that was Thatcherism (Gamble 1988, Jessop *et al.* 1988). The demand-led nature of general practice services brought about escalating expenditure, which posed a considerable challenge to the general policies of retrenchment practised in the 1980s. To this end, common themes were value for money, marketisation and choice, and regulation and responsibility.

The first precursor theme has already been noted. General management introduced a challenge to medical power and a culture of competition and performance. While the Griffiths management inquiry had prescribed general management as a treatment for all the NHS (DHSS 1983), its impact was felt most directly in the hospital and community health services. Superficially, primary care remained relatively unaffected. Nevertheless, the emergence of general management brought about marked indirect changes in promoting the idea of managed services. This shift in emphasis can be argued to have had profound long-term consequences for primary care and general practice, underpinning the increased role of non-medical practice managers and the position of general practice as an integrated element in the overall management of the NHS.

The initial stages of this process were both facilitated and evidenced by the small NHS reorganisation which came into effect on 1 April 1985. It was on that date that FPCs ceased to be simply the bodies that arranged the remuneration of GPs and other primary care service providers. They took on responsibilities for the planning and development of primary care and were expected to collaborate with district health authorities and local authorities over joint service planning across the health and social care interface. In taking on these managerial tasks, FPCs were able to begin setting limits on the autonomy of the individual general practice. It was, in practice, to be some years before this was to have any real impact. The FPCs of the late 1980s often remained consensual administrative bodies rather than overt managers of general practice services. Arguably it was only with the demise in the mid-1990s of the FPCs' successors, the Family Health Services Authorities (FHSAs), that the basis for a managed service could really be said to have been constructed; 1985 was, however, the year in which the process began.

The second precursor theme was centrally concerned with GP pharmaceutical prescribing, a key element in the escalating costs of the general practice service. This was a problematic issue as GPs had traditionally had the clinical freedom to prescribe whichever drugs they deemed appropriate in whatever quantity; within families of drugs with similar effects, there was no compulsion to select the most economic therapy. The result of this freedom was an inability on the part of government to control GP prescribing behaviour, and the consequent and continuing financial implications. The idea of a limited drug list, first floated in 1984, was intended to constrain GPs to the prescription of drugs that an expert panel had decided achieved the required therapeutic goal at the lowest cost. The proposal was greeted with trenchant opposition from the BMA and the pharmaceutical industry. This opposition led to some modifications. Some brand-name formulations were to be abandoned in favour of more generic preparations and, in a foretaste of later stresses on prescribing economics and evidence-based medicine, there was a particular focus on linking effectiveness and economy, most notably in the prescribing of common respiratory and decongestant medicines. Drug costs were to be further reduced by structured negotiations between the NHS and the pharmaceutical industry.

Ham (1992a) claims that the introduction of the limited list saved the NHS £75 million in the first year during which the policy operated. Its implementation was accompanied by year-on-year annual rises in prescription charges. Subsequent development saw the provision to practices of progressively more detailed information on their prescribing via the introduction in 1988 of the prescribing analysis and costs system (PACT) and, after *Working for Patients* (DoH 1989a), indicative drug budgets and comparative prescribing data. The limited list was thus, like the creation of the FPCs, an indication of a trend that was to be accentuated in the future. It showed that it was possible to develop, against hard opposition, a legislative framework that could curb GP behaviour even in the face of allegations of offences against clinical freedom.

The ideas that general practice might be managed and that GP autonomy might be curbed were therefore established items on the NHS agenda prior to the White Paper. What though of the practical focus of the White Paper? As will be seen below, it placed great stress on the promotion of good health and the prevention of premature mortality. This emphasis constitutes the third area in which a substantial foundation for the measures in the White Paper had already been laid. In the late 1970s, Old Labour had produced a discussion document and a White Paper (DHSS 1976a, 1977) that had firmly linked the possibility of further improvements in collective health status to the need for individuals to take responsibility for their own health and choose healthy lifestyles. Their argument was that major strides in health status had been achieved by public health measures and, to a far lesser extent, by medical intervention. Any more improvement was down to individual actions. These notions of choice, responsibility and individualism were attractive to the Conservative Party of the 1980s. It was therefore not perhaps surprising that the primary care White Paper made great play of health promotion (Williams *et al.* 1993), nor that it delivered that emphasis within a context in which preventive services were simultaneously offered to the public on a voluntary basis while GPs were regulated and rewarded on the basis of their success in meeting specified performance targets.

The Green Paper

For Wilkin *et al.* (1987:5), the Green Paper *Primary Health Care: An Agenda for Discussion* (DHSS 1986b) was the essential beginning of the process of constructing general practice as part of the managed NHS. It was 'the first attempt to carry out a comprehensive review of primary health care'. In terms of content, it was strongly and unsurprisingly dominated by the then current Conservative belief in the effectiveness of market forces as a basis for the production of quality public services. Equally unsurprising, given the size of the Conservative parliamentary majority, was the survival of its recommendations, largely intact, as the foundation for the subsequent White Paper. Yet some minor wonder, if not outright surprise, must be registered at this survival. The changes proposed were fundamental and challenged a powerful popular constituency. In no small part, the ability of the Conservative government to propose and then implement its recommendations concerning primary care constituted a foretaste of its strategy and success with its wider programme of NHS reform some four years later.

Incentives were central to the Green Paper. It recommended the institution of a 'good-practice allowance' that would reward those GPs who provided good services. This was explicitly an attempt to use market mechanisms and financial reward as a means of raising the quality of general practice. A particular emphasis was placed on ensuring the delivery of quality services in inner city environments, where an inquiry had recently revealed significant problems in primary care delivery (see Chapter 7). 'Good services' and 'quality services' were conceptualised by reference to two themes.

First, they were seen as being inherently orientated towards the prevention of ill-health and disease. Screening, either opportunistically during routine consultations in the surgery, or via a more structured process outlining requirements to screen defined fractions of the population for specified conditions, was heavily promoted. Target payments were proposed for the latter form of activity.

The second principle underlying ideas on service quality concerned the provider of care, the GP. The Green Paper sought to ensure that GPs and general practice would be as widely available as possible, with service hours clearly publicised and sufficiently extensive to safeguard rights of access on the part of the general public. It also set out a specification for GP continuing education intended to secure, for the public, a reasonable guarantee that GPs would be aware of current advances in medical science. These aspects of the Green Paper were to be delivered by the payment of education allowances and a requirement for much greater levels of publicity concerning general practice hours and services.

The theme of quality was also extended in other ways. It was suggested that GPs might face compulsory retirement at 70. This proposal was intended to address the option that GPs then had of 'retiring' for one day and then returning to continue in practice until whenever they wished to retire. Although evidence was never wholly conclusive, and numerous exceptions existed, there were suggestions that older GPs tended to be less likely to practise preventive medicine and more likely to follow reactive strategies, prescribe more but less effectively, work from less satisfactory premises and be available less frequently (LHPC 1981).

It was also proposed that the make-up of GP remuneration should be changed. The basic practice allowance, the allowance payable simply for operating a general practice, was felt to lack the capacity to incentivise GPs. Its salience in remuneration was to be reduced in favour of an increased capitation element reflecting the size of the general practice. The Green Paper was careful, however, not to imply a simplistic link between list size and quality of care. Instead, the intention was to reward GPs who were able to attract more patients and recognise that the provision of good care to a larger number of people was inherently likely to incur greater costs.

There were also to be other measures concerned with information provision. Practice reports and practice leaflets were proposed. These were intended to make it easier for the public to know what was being done in general practice and also to facilitate choice. As a by-product of this stress on choice, it was also recognised that people should be able to change their GP more easily and that GPs themselves needed better information on their activities. With regard to the former issue, it was proposed that patients should no longer need the permission of the GP whom they were leaving. Proposals with respect to the latter focused on the provision of information about drug prescribing, with a subtext on the promotion of more rational prescribing following on from the issues noted earlier in the chapter. There were also suggestions that GPs might be provided with comparative information on their rates of referral to secondary care, although it was acknowledged that these would need to be adjusted to reflect differences in case mix (variations in disease incidence and severity between GPs).

There was one further proposal in the Green Paper that merits a mention. 'Health care shops' were to be one-stop locations where people would find all forms of primary health care and some follow-up care available under one roof. Private and public sector providers were to co-exist and co-refer, funding being provided on a capitation basis. This proposal was undoubtedly innovative. It breached the notion of the NHS as a (largely) public sector operation and sought a level of integration between sectors and between types of service that was far beyond anything then currently existing in the UK. Parallels elsewhere were imperfect. The idea owed something to the health maintenance organisations (HMOs) then beginning to attract significant attention in the USA (see Chapter 10). They also, perhaps strangely given the politics of the time, bore some similarity to the polyclinics that characterised health care provision in the socialist health care systems. Interestingly, many developments such as total purchasing and primary care trusts, which emerged in the last years of Conservative government in the mid-1990s or later under New Labour pursued the same goals of integration and collaboration.

The reaction to the Green Paper was mixed. The RCGP (1987) criticised the increased proportion of its members' incomes that was expected to be derived from capitation fees. These threatened, in its eyes, to generate competition between GPs and lead to ever larger lists in the quest for income maximisation, and hence to reduced attention for the individual patient. The forcefulness of this opposition was somewhat tempered, however, by the impact of earlier RCGP work, which had argued that the enhancement of the quality of general practice care demanded action on many of the proposals set out in the Green Paper, including targets and incentives (RCGP 1985). Wilkin *et al.* (1987:135) offered a more ideological critique. The Green Paper, they suggested, demonstrated a 'misplaced faith in the effectiveness of market forces'. On the other hand, the Association of Community Health Councils welcomed the Green Paper for its proposed commitment to a more open regulation of the primary care sector despite its arguably over-heavy focus on general practice at the expense of other elements of the primary care team (ACHCEW 1986).

The White Paper

As suggested above, much of the primary care Green Paper subsequently appeared in the White Paper *Promoting Better Health* (DHSS 1987). The White Paper itself 'signified a major turning point regarding not only the issue of prevention, but also the place and function of primary health care within the NHS' (Williams *et al.* 1993:44). Its aims were to make services more responsive to the consumer, to raise standards of care, to promote health and prevent illness, to give patients the widest range of choice in obtaining high-quality primary care services, to improve value for money and to enable clearer priorities to be set for FPSs in relation to the rest of the health service (DHSS 1987). The actions arising from these aims are summarised in Table 3.1.

The White Paper made it clear that competition and performance were now acceptable aspects of general practice (Powell 1997). It stated that 'no

Table 3.1   General practice and the White Paper *Promoting Better Health* (DHSS 1987): aims and key measures

Aims	Measures
Consumer responsiveness	Easier to change GP
Consumer choice	Easier to complain about GP More information about general practices Incentives to practise in deprived or rural areas
Raising standards of care	GPs to retire at 70 Postgraduate Education Allowance Allow growth of primary health care team (but cash limited)
Health promotion	Target payments for immunisation and screening
Disease prevention	Health checks on new patients and the elderly Payments for minor surgery Health promotion clinics
Improved value for money	Increased proportion of GP income from capitation payments Stiffened eligibility for Basic Practice Allowance
Clarify role of Family Practitioner Services	FPCs get more control over regulation and resourcing FPCs agree targets and monitor them FPCs increase surveillance of prescribing
Other	Encouragement of computerisation Dental and optician charges

FPC = Family Practitioner Committee.

opportunity should be lost to increase fair and open competition between those providing family practitioner services. To that end... the remuneration of practitioners should be more directly linked than at present to the level of their performance' (DHSS 1987). Choice was also to be facilitated. Patients who wanted to change their GP would be assisted and helped in that process. Barriers to change that had placed the control of this process with the GP were to be reduced. The expected consequence of this process was that public choice would reveal more popular GPs, and that those who proved less popular would find their capitation-based incomes reduced and thus have an incentive to improve the quality of their service. To aid this process further, the proportion of GPs' incomes derived from capitation payments was to be raised from 46 to 60 per cent (Ham 1992a).

Changes were also proposed to other aspects of GP remuneration. GPs who performed better were to be rewarded with more money. Performance targets were set in a number of areas, most notably screening and childhood immunisation, and payments were instituted for reaching the targets. There were also to be rewards for health promotion work: fees became payable for offering screening to older patients and people joining a practice. Minor surgery in general practices was facilitated, and specific allowances were put in place to reward GPs practising in areas of high deprivation or rural isola- tion. It was noted that 'some doctors appear to do no more than the minimum requirement', so the then current basic practice allowance (see above) of £7,850 for at least 1,000 patients and 20 hours of direct services was the subject of significant adjustment. Both the patient and the availability param- eters were increased, and it was made a requirement that GPs undertook health promotion activity (Baggott 1994).

Within general practices, there was an encouragement of computerisation, aiming to improve information flow, facilitate streamlined administration and enable planned rather than reactive care. Restrictions were also removed on the number and type of staff who could be employed by GPs as part of the primary health care team. Neither computerisation nor the removal of staffing restrictions was without problems. The former engendered consider- able competition among software suppliers, many linked to pharmaceutical companies. The result was the emergence in general practice of a multiplicity of different computer systems and consequent communication and support difficulties, which only began to resolve over a decade later. The removal of staffing restrictions brought general practice into conflict with other parts of the NHS over the employment of nurses able to work outside hospital settings. Baggott (1994) reports how the number of practice nurses, for example, doubled from 5,000 to 10,000 in the two years from 1988 to 1990. In a situation of a perennial crisis of nursing staff level, this growth inevitably occurred at the expense of other parts of the NHS.

Further measures saw the creation of targeted improvement grants for surgeries in poor repair and the promise of a review of minimum standards for surgery provision. The use of private finance to enable improvements was also encouraged. Patients, clearly seen as the 'consumers' of a service, were to be given greater information on opening hours and on practices. Practices were to be required to produce annual reports. Changing GP was made easier, the requirement for permission to leave a GP being abolished. Complaints mechanisms were also streamlined, with oral complaints being allowed and the window for complaint being extended to 13 weeks. Finally, there was to be encouragement to women entrants to general practice and to part-time GPs, regular postgraduate education was to be the subject of financial incentive, and the retirement age was fixed at 70.

There were three areas broached in the Green Paper that did not make it to the White Paper. The 'good-practice allowance' was not introduced as such. The intentions of the proposal were, however, implicitly present in the various incentives and target payments set out in *Promoting Better Health*. The stiffer eligibility criteria for the basic practice allowance also worked in the spirit of the good-practice allowance. In essence, therefore, a series of measures replaced one single proposal. This had the merit of offering the possibility of enhanced income and performance assessment across a range of factors while at the same time avoiding an overt separation of the good from the bad, which would have been more offensive to the GP population. The second proposal that failed to make the White Paper was the one on health care shops. It is probable that the organisational costs of this proposal were felt to outweigh the potential gains; elements of private sector input were, however, facilitated by the encouragement of private finance for loans for the improvement of surgery premises.

Proposals for more realistic prescription charges were the third omission. This had consequences for the size of the fiscal base needed to pay for the reforms, reforms that were also to generate significant new costs in terms of the proposed incentive payments to GPs for health promotion work. Although a much tighter monitoring of prescribing was instituted, a further injection of cash was needed. Even though, in the event, it proved wholly inadequate, this need was addressed by a major proposal that lay outside the immediate area of concern of general practice. It was recommended that charging arrangements be introduced for eye tests and dental check-ups. The latter charges were in addition to existing charges for the costs of dental treatment, which were themselves to be raised to 75 per cent of the total real costs of treatment.

The effect of both these changes was to diminish the extent to which the NHS could truly be seen as a service free to the consumer at the point of contact. Their introduction effectively ended free eye care within the NHS for all but certain exempt categories of patient (Timmins 1988:56). They also indirectly hastened the decline of NHS dentistry. Charges discouraged service uptake, particularly among those sectors of society least able to afford the new charges. As a consequence, in the longer term, there were negative effects on oral health, and general dental practitioners, working increasingly with more affluent population groups, found the attractions of a more substantially private sector mode of organisation less bureaucratically demanding and financially more attractive. It is ironic, as Powell (1997:121) remarks, 'that these policies had their roots in a document entitled "Promoting Better Health". Here was an action in which there was a clear contrast between the rhetoric of subscribing to the principle that "prevention is better than cure" and applying it in practice.'

Despite the fact that its impact on dental and optician services was therefore far-reaching, the main substance of *Promoting Better Health* was concerned with general practice. This was unsurprising given the dominant position of GP services in primary health care, as noted in Chapter 1. It was, however, an inevitable basis for criticism of the White Paper. As Marks (1989:1) remarked, '[it has] done little to promote a strategic policy for primary care as a whole'. In focusing on FPSs and, within that category, largely on GP services, the White Paper had taken a narrow definition of primary care, one which rested on the agency of experts and lacked the consumer/patient input that would have characterised an approach more in tune with WHO perspectives (1978). The argument that the White Paper was essentially a medicalised response to the need for reforms in the primary care arena also underpinned suggestions that the focus on general practice and the GP as the basis for the development of incentives was an implicit undervaluing of the crucial contributions that other professional groups would make to the achievement of targets and indicative of an overoptimistic reliance on the abilities of GPs to adjust their behaviour towards a more preventive orientation. In short, the criticism was that GPs would reap the benefits while other professional groups, notably health visitors and practice nurses, undertook the work. GPs would also find it difficult to shift their practice towards population-based services such as screening and away from opportunistic individual care.

A second group of criticisms focused on the probable implementation difficulties that it was thought the White Paper would bring. Above all, these were seen in terms of the workload implications. GPs were certainly to be rewarded for undertaking extra activities, but those activities were definitely additional to what was commonly on offer in general practice. Furthermore, information and reporting requirements were being much extended; this too would bring extra work. Such increases in workload were, it was argued, likely to detract from the business of providing direct patient care (RCGP 1987). The temptation might have been to oppose or even not cooperate with the reforms. However, as Calnan and Gabe note, 'Evaluating the performance of GPs is in line with the state's policy of attempting to limit the autonomy of certain professional groups. The White Paper makes it clear that if GPs do not monitor the quality of their performance, then they are at risk that the state will do it for them' (Calnan and Gabe 1991:152). In the event, the extra work-load was largely met by appointing additional staff, both clinical and managerial. The 'paperwork' burden in general practice was, however, to remain as a running grievance.

The final group of criticisms that can be levelled at *Promoting Better Health* concern the strengthening of the FPC role. It was accepted that this was necessary by all but the most extreme advocates of GP autonomy. For example, Allsop and May (1986) had very clearly identified the inability of the FPCs to deliver on the extended managerial and planning role that they had been given in 1985. Their undeniably economical operation in fact hid considerable underresourcing. This, combined with difficulties dealing with powerful, autonomous GPs and a lack of liaison with district health authori-ties, was limiting their future ability to develop a strategic direction to primary care (NAO 1988). In *Promoting Better Health* the government recog-nised the substantial progress that FPCs had made within these constraints, but it was made clear that there would need to be further developments.

The 1990 GP Contract

The proposals set out in the primary care White Paper were, with respect to general medical practice, largely implemented through the 1990 GP contract (GB Departments of Health 1989). This contract made substantial changes to the terms of employment of GPs, as well as to their remuneration. It was the subject of lengthy negotiation with the profession but was not ratified. On being circulated in 1989, it was stated that 'The package of changes set out in this document takes account of the views expressed by the negotiators during the consultation and the government believes that the package forms a sound basis for a new contract between GPs and the NHS' (GB Departments of Health 1989:1). The package became operative on 1 April 1990.

The 1990 contract replaced the 1965/66 contract that had been created as part of the Family Doctors' Charter (Chapter 2). That earlier contract had also been presented in the spirit of an ultimatum (Loudon *et al.* 1998), although opposition had been far less trenchant and the basis for acceptance by the profession was in fact in place. In operation, the 1965/66 contract had proved both durable and popular. There were two aspects to the 1965/66 contract that the 1990 contract was to alter substantially. First, the earlier contract had, to an extent, moved GP remuneration away from a system to which the 1990 contract now proposed a return. A substantial part of the GP's income before 1965 had come from a capitation fee. The 1965/66 contract introduced and gave equal prominence to the basic practice allowance. Second, the various 'supplements' to the basic practice allowance were paid largely as allowances rather than by reference to any targets or strategic direction.

The context for the implementation of the 1990 contract was that of the reformed NHS as set out in *Working for Patients* (DoH 1989a). FPCs had been superseded by FHSAs. The FPCs had relied on a professional ethos and had been led by a committee on which there had been eight GPs. FHSAs, in contrast, had to have just one GP member. They were also accountable to regional health authorities alongside district health authorities, rather than being accountable only to central government. FHSAs had enhanced responsibilities and could exert enhanced control (DoH 1990). They regulated and targeted cash-limited budgets for premises, staff and drugs, and were charged with bringing the gains from the wider NHS reform agenda into the primary care sector. From April 1991, this changed operational environment also featured GP fundholders (see Chapter 4). On top of the demands of the new contract, these latter GPs also had a budget for the direct purchase of secondary care.

The content of the contract was essentially a replication of the themes that had been emerging through the Green and White Papers and even before. Table 3.2 summarises the key developments, focusing on the issue of remuneration to GPs. The contract consultation document admirably summarised the governmental perspectives underpinning the new system:

> Value for money is now an essential ingredient in all areas of public expenditure and performance related pay is a common feature in many public sector remuneration systems. Greater competition in the provision of services is now a major feature in both private and public enterprise because it encourages a better service to consumers. (DoH/Welsh Office, 1989:28)

Four main criticisms of the new GP contract can be identified. First, in emphasising capitation, it exposed GPs to the volatility of patient choice. For the government, this was the market in operation. For GPs, however, it was arguably lacking in sensitivity concerning the potential financial implications. Making it easier to change doctors was seen as encouraging doctor-swapping without necessarily good cause. Some GPs might, as a consequence, go out of business. Others, running popular practices, might be swamped with excess demand (Leavey *et al.* 1989). Second, as already noted, the financial rewards of the new contract were to be achieved only at the expense of a considerably enhanced workload in terms of both activities and the associated regulatory and claim procedures. Furthermore, the acceptance of this increased workload was often either unavoidable or simply a matter of economic necessity. Practices were, for example, loath to refuse to run services offered by their local 'competitors' or to set out figures in their annual reports indicating a failure to

Table 3.2 Proposed GP remuneration in the 1990 contract

Fee element	Comments
Capitation	• To equate to 60% of GP income • Absorbs seniority and group practice allowances • Enhanced for under-5s, over-75s and new patient populations provided health checks are provided
Basic practice allowance	• Reduced element of GP income; converted to a capitation payment • Payable for first 1,500 patients • Not payable to GPs with fewer than 500 patients • Enhanced to reflect patient number in deprived areas • Enhanced to reflect patient number in sparsely populated areas
Training allowance	• Allowance for continuing education concerning health promotion, disease management and service management • Payable on presentation of evidence of attendance at accredited courses to a specified annual amount averaged over five years
Target payments	• Payment for achieving 90% coverage for childhood immunisations • Payment for achieving 80% coverage for cervical cytology
Health promotion	• Sessional fee for well-person, diabetes, heart disease, anti-smoking, stress management and alcohol control clinics. Other clinics at FHSA discretion • Health checks every three years for the adult population
Other	• Allowance for teaching undergraduate medical students • Sessional fee for specified minor surgery procedures assuming one session per month • Isolation payment for single-handed, remote rural GPs • Continuation of night visit fees

N.B. Some proposals were later modified, for example lower level target payments being added for immunisation (70%) and cervical cytology (50%).
FHSA = Family Health Services Authority.

meet targets for immunisation or screening. Third, there was concern that tactically minded GPs would artificially adjust their practice populations by refusing to accept new patients who would damage their chances of meeting targets or generating extra income from allowances. Finally, there was doubt about the clinical effectiveness of some of the proposed requirements, particularly the requirements to screen new patients and all patients at three-year intervals (Waller *et al.* 1990). These doubts would continue as evidence-based health care emerged during the 1990s and centred on the dangers of devoting excess time to screening the well. McIntyre *et al.* (1992), evaluating patients' knowledge of changes to GP services six months after implementation of the 1990 contract, found that the public shared professionals' doubts about the effectiveness of these measures. It was this last criticism that was to be the subject of specific attention in the 1993 review of the contract (GMSC 1993).

Promotion and Prevention: Case Studies

Having now identified the considerable stress placed on health promotion and disease prevention in general practice settings by the primary health care reforms of the 1980s, and analysed the context in which this emphasis emerged, our attention turns to three case studies. These have been selected in order to draw upon research evidence of the operation of the measures identified in the 1990 GP contract. They are: health promotion clinics, health check screening, and target payments for childhood immunisation.

Health Promotion Clinics

The 1990 contract saw an amendment to GPs' terms of service to include an obligation to provide health promotion services to the non-elderly adult population. This population was defined as people aged between 16 and 74. There were three ways in which health promotion services could be provided: opportunistically during contacts or consultations initiated by the patient, by invitation to special consultations for patients not seen within the past three years, or via sessions at clinics specially set up to cover health promotion themes. The introduction of funded health promotion clinics was seen as 'something of a surprise [which] becomes an unusual area of innovation and expansion in the primary care sector' (Yen 1995:26). Accordingly, it is on this topic that this subsection focuses.

General practices running health promotion clinics could apply for support funds from their FHSA. The GP who organised the clinic was rewarded with a fixed fee of £45. To access these funds, they had to hold a clinic for 10 people on a health promotion topic agreed with the FHSA. An indicative list of topics included 'wellness', diabetes, alcohol misuse, smoking cessation, heart health, diet control and stress management. The relatively open-ended nature of the permissible content of health promotion clinics and the absence of cash limitations on the initiative ensured that there was a proliferation of small clinics. There was no need for practices to compete for resources. Indeed, for general practice, it was sound business sense to extend the range of services provided from the practice base.

The expansion of health promotion clinics in general practice was further fuelled by pressures elsewhere in the NHS. Although it was the GP organising the clinic who was rewarded with a fixed fee, most health promotion clinics were staffed not by GPs themselves or even by practice staff, but by employees of NHS provider units. The effects of the implementation of the internal market alongside the implementation of the GP contract ensured that trusts were actively looking for markets for their health promotion services at the same time as GPs were actively looking for people to provide health promotion services. The need for trusts to build their businesses coincided well with GP need. In cases where trusts were unable to satisfy GP demands, a burgeoning private health promotion industry was also able to contribute to the growth in the number of clinics.

Given the essentially unplanned nature of the growth of GP health promotion clinics, it is no surprise that what was provided often bore little relationship to need. Most GPs had a relatively rudimentary knowledge of health promotion at the time, and their views were often shaped by clinical priorities and a medical rather than social perspective; the holistic social approach of health promotion sat uncomfortably alongside more traditional notions of illness management. For example, Coulter and Schofield (1991), in a study of 1,014 GPs in the Oxford Region, found that attitudes to prevention and health promotion were very positive, but few respondents made a point of discussing smoking habits (64 per cent), alcohol intake (26 per cent), diet (12 per cent) or exercise (11 per cent) as a matter of routine with their adult patients, and most GPs usually offered only simple advice, leaflets or other aids when they identified a problem. Bruce and Burnett (1991) further noted caution on the part of GPs concerning their effectiveness as health promoters, the real likelihood of achieving change, their ability to cope with the anticipated workload and its conflict with curative work.

As a consequence of these factors, many of the clinics set up under the framework of the contract were not really concerned with health promotion at all. Some sought to build links between allopathic medicine and therapies such as chiropody and physiotherapy. Others were concerned with chronic illness management and not necessarily only with diabetes care. Still further clinics focused on very specific needs such as sports medicine. The central role of the GP in determining what clinics were to be set up under the rubric of health promotion ensured that clinic take-up was usually by referral from the GP. Clinics were seldom accessed directly by the public or even used by people who were not frequent attenders at the practice. Had it not been for the subsidy, many clinics would have been uneconomic to run. Nevertheless, they broadened the base of general practice, and, in extending the range of services provided from GP premises, the centrality of the GP in health care delivery was ensured across a canvas far broader than that traditionally occupied by general medical practice.

Gillam (1992) explored the implementation of health promotion clinics across one family health services authority. Single-handed practices were less likely to be running health promotion clinics. The concentration of such practices in deprived wards with historically high mortality rates meant that practices located in wards where the standardised mortality ratio was greater than 100, and practices receiving deprivation payments, were less likely to be offering health promotion clinics. This finding implied the relevance of the inverse care law to the provision of health promotion clinics. While begging the question of the effectiveness of health promotion clinics, provision tended to ignore populations at higher risk of ill-health.

McMahon and Bodansky (1991), in their discussion of the intentions of GPs in Leeds (UK) towards diabetes care, make a further point. Although 76 per cent of practices expressed an interest in starting a diabetic clinic, facilities in many were lacking, and less than half could offer in-practice access to complementary services such as chiropody and dietetic advice. Some expertise in diabetes was claimed by only 10 (22 per cent) doctors, and staff at all practices identified a need for further training. The economic imperative of health promotion often lacked a sound base in expertise.

By 1991/92 health promotion clinics were something of a 'must-have' accessory in general practice. They certainly assisted practices in competing against each other. On the other hand, however, they had drawn staff away from other parts of the NHS. They had had a particular impact on staffing levels in the professions allied to medicine, notably physiotherapy. This had taken staff away from areas with a demonstrable effectiveness, such as stroke rehabilitation, and moved them to areas where effectiveness in terms of outcome had yet to be demonstrated. The lack of control over expenditure had fuelled an unfettered user-responsiveness. In some extreme cases, clinics had been set up in areas such as body enhancement that might more properly have been seen as appropriate for the private sector.

The 1993 amendment to the GP contract (GMSC 1993) sought to curb these excesses and rein in the unmanaged development of health promotion in general practice. It spelled the end of the individualised free market approach to health promotion and facilitated a move towards a managed market in which programmes of activities could be identified and targeted on risk management in populations. To this end, it could be argued that it represented a further extension of the process of moving GPs away from a simple concern with the health of the consulting population towards an involvement in the health of the whole of their list population, both consulters and non-consulters.

The Health of the Nation White Paper (DoH 1992a), the first attempt in England at a national health, as opposed to health care, policy, provided the context for the 1993 contract amendment as far as health promotion was concerned. Health promotion was recentred on the identification and targeting of risk with regard to the topic areas singled out in *The Health of the Nation* document. A particular stress was placed on combating coronary heart disease and stroke within the practice population. Following the lead set in *The Health of the Nation* White Paper, the approach to health promotion was strongly biomedical. There was an emphasis on measurement and the quantification of risk.

The 1990 contract had required the recording of smoking, blood pressure, weight, drinking and family histories of disease; the 1993 amendment explicitly sought outreach on the part of the GP. There was to be an expectation of 90 per cent practice coverage for blood pressure recording, 80 per cent for smoking status and 75 per cent for body mass, alcohol use and family history. Three bands or levels of activity were set (GMSC 1993, NHSE 1993). The top band involved information collection, risk identification and analysis, and intervention aimed at heart disease and stroke. Existing clinics had to be repackaged to fit with the new system or abandoned; some of the more esoteric provision was privatised. Alongside coronary heart disease and stroke, only the disease-specific areas of diabetes care and asthma control were retained as acceptable bases for health promotion and disease prevention clinics.

The 1993 contract provided a structure and framework for the development of health promotion clinics in general practice. It sought focused coverage at the population level and worked from an evidence base rather than being led by whim and economic opportunism. In instituting control, however, it also brought increased reporting burdens. Nevertheless, band three health promotion applications were common, and it appears that most GPs were willing to trade off the loss of autonomy for a more structured approach to health promotion.

Health Check Screening

Yen (1995) argues that the 1990 GP contract introduced an approach to health promotion that commodified that activity and encouraged patients to make choices for health. This was particularly evident in the voluntaristic nature of certain aspects of the health promotion package. While GPs were expected to *offer* services, the public could *choose* whether to take up their offer. Responsible GPs would ensure an attractive offer; responsible members of a patient list would wish to look after their own health and would thus take up the offer. This approach was, as already noted above, applied to the 'health check screening' of people on a GP list aged between 16 and 74 who had not been seen during the previous three years. It was also applied annually to all people aged over 75.

Superficially, health check screening appears to be a good idea. It should provide baseline information on patients and demonstrate the GP's commitment to ensuring an awareness of the health needs of all people on her or his list. Whether undertaken opportunistically or using more structured means, the offer of a health check should show that the GP cares. It also makes sound use of the unique access that GPs have to the population. Most of the population are registered with a GP and, as *Promoting Better Health* noted, 'Through their regular contact with families and patients, family doctors... are well-placed to promote good health and to prevent ill-health by giving advice on lifestyle [and] by providing screening' (DHSS 1987:13). More critically, however, health checks can also be seen as unnecessary surveillance conducted with no clear end in mind, no specific targets, no guidelines for action and no intention to aggregate the information for profiling purposes or to share with other agencies.

This critical perspective is particularly evident with regard to the requirement to offer general health checks to the adult population. Morris *et al.* (1992) reviewed consultation rates over a period of three years for 7,010 middle-aged men. They compared the cardio-respiratory health and risk factor status of non-consulters (men who did not consult in three years) with those of average consulters (men who consulted 3–5 times in three years) and high consulters (men who consulted 24 or more times in three years) to assess their relative need for health promotion and illness prevention services. The non-consulters were remarkably similar to the average consulters in health and lifestyle characteristics. The high consulters had a greater burden of ill-health and a less healthy lifestyle. From this, Morris *et al.* concluded that most health problems were already known to GPs and that screening non-consulters would reveal little hidden morbidity. Noakes (1991) drew similar conclusions suggesting that 'no particular evidence is apparent which should deflect general practice from its present opportunistic approach to screening'. A small study by Thompson (1990) went further. A total of 114 patients who had not attended their GP in the previous three years were identified, and an invitation for a health check was sent. Seventeen attended. The group responding to the invitation were in general healthy, and the smoking rate and alcohol consumption rate were low. One new case of mild hypertension was found. Of 13 patients who needed a tetanus immunisation, five refused it and five failed to return. All three women who were overdue for a cervical smear failed to return. Surgery staff spent 28 hours, and the practice doctors spent 15 hours, arranging and carrying out the screening. Thompson concluded that three-year health checks were not an efficient use of medical time. Quantitatively, this would appear to be the case, although caution should be exercised in generalising from such a small study, and it would perhaps be more relevant to note the hidden health care need that was revealed.

A better case can be made for health check screening for people aged over 75. Perkins (1991) argued that although the new contract disregards much of the medical research, there are benefits to be gained. Brown *et al.* (1992) provide a sound evaluation of elderly screening in operation in one FHSA. Visits were made to 20 general practices to collect information on how assessments were organised and carried out. The way in which health checks were performed varied greatly. Three practices had not performed any checks. Thirteen practices sent a letter to invite patients to undergo a check. Of these practices, seven followed up non-responders. Many old people did not respond to the letter asking whether they wanted an assessment, but very few refused one if followed up. Two practices visited patients' homes unannounced, and two carried out checks only on an opportunistic basis. Forty-three per cent of those assessed had some unmet need. In one sample month, 204 new problems were discovered, significantly more per patient being found in inner city areas. These findings again point to the resource implications of screening in terms of the extra problems that it identifies. They also indicate that most unmet need may fall in high-risk areas.

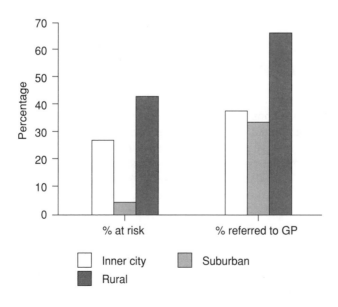

Figure 3.1 Spatial variations in elderly screening

Figure 3.1 substantiates these points. It is drawn from a study conducted in a large health authority in southern England. The first set of columns considers the issue of risk and isolates the more severe health problems uncovered by screening. Following Brown *et al.* (1992), there are clearly more at-risk older people in inner city environments than in more affluent suburban areas. There are, however, even more at risk in rural communities, where risk may be partially formed by problems of physical isolation from services. The second column in the figure indicates the implications of screening for GP workload. Notwithstanding variations in risk, there are broadly similar levels of implication for GP workload in inner city and suburban locations. In rural areas, a follow-up consultation with the GP is by far the most common outcome of a screening.

What is not evident in Figure 3.1 or in the discussion of other studies is the scope for operator variation in screening. Notwithstanding different approaches to 'offering' screening, screening, when taken up, can also be delivered in different ways. Most simply, one screener's 'risk' can result in a referral, while for another it may be an acceptable part of life. No consensus has emerged on what exactly should be done or on guidelines for follow-up action. This lack of uniformity means that some elderly people inevitably miss out on potential benefits, while others, the worried well, might be argued to consume scarce resources unnecessarily. The need to respect the autonomy of GPs and the confidentiality of the doctor–patient consultation ensures that this variation is likely to persist.

Immunisation Targets

The 1990 contract replaced fee-for-service payments for cervical cytology and childhood immunisation with a system of payments linked to target levels of uptake (Chisholm 1990). In this way, performance was explicitly linked to remuneration. A comparison of relative performances was expected to lead to improvements on the part of those practices with lower levels of uptake (Allen *et al.* 1987, Newlands and Davies 1988), the underlying aim being to develop general practice through the improvement of services to patients (Bain 1990).

The target level of uptake for childhood immunisations was initially set at 90 per cent of the practice list population of children who reached the age of two during the year preceding the claim, this being the WHO's recommended target uptake. The achievement of the target entailed the completion of a complete series of immunisations for diphtheria, tetanus and pertussis (DTP), poliomyelitis and measles (subsequently measles, mumps and rubella [MMR]). To some considerable extent, this target was eminently achievable; uptake rates were generally at or around 90 per cent by the time of the contract. The exceptions to this generality were the pertussis element of the DTP triple vaccine, which had yet to recover from adverse publicity concerning a raised risk of side-effects (Nichol 1985) and, to a lesser extent, measles immunisation. A lower uptake for these immunisations could depress the overall uptake and, as a consequence, a lower target of 70 per cent was also put in place and linked to a lower level of reward. No payments were to be made to practices failing to reach the lower target.

Jones *et al.* (1992) note how the achievement of an immunisation target reflects processes operating at two different levels. First, there are factors associated with the exercise of choice and the effects of constraint on a child's parent(s). New and Senior (1992) cite gender role constraints under this heading. Mothers usually act as prime carers and decision-makers concerning childhood immunisations. They are less likely to attend for an immunisation if they have other small children or lack educational qualifications. A classic panoply of indicators of social deprivation was also linked to failure to immunise. These included overcrowding, local authority housing tenure, high population mobility, lower social class and the membership of a minority ethnic group (McIntosh *et al.* 1981, Marsh and Channing 1986, Bhopal and Samin 1988, Jarman *et al.* 1988, Peckham 1989). A second group of factors related to the general practice and concerned the quality of recall systems and the knowledge base of the GP. At this level, there were also indications that smaller practices with older GPs were less likely to return a high uptake rate (Jarman *et al.* 1988).

The sum effect of these processes was that uptake rates at the time of the introduction of the contract were subject to some considerable geographical variation, reflecting both the composition of practice child populations and the varying contextual characteristics of practices. When (and where) particular combinations of contextual and compositional factors coincided, the level of uptake could be much lower than average. Leese and Bosanquet (1992), for example, contended that inner city areas (and practices) had particularly low levels of childhood immunisation. Jones *et al.* (1992) summarised this situation thus: 'both "who you are" – the client characteristics – and "where you go" – the practice factors – are important in determining uptake'. In a companion paper, Jones and Moon (1991) went on to note that: 'Given a list dominated by patients with characteristics known to be associated with low uptake, some practices "perform" well yet have low uptakes... practices that are effective with low uptake groups may provide models of good practice.' They also challenged the wisdom of basing payments on crude percentage uptake measures that would probably be vulnerable to considerable fluctuation in the case of practices with a low base number of children.

A multilevel modelling approach allowed Jones and Moon (1991) to take account of both the base number problem and the interplay of composition and context. Multilevel models allow a separate consideration of influences

Table 3.3   Contextualising immunisation uptake performance: the 10 best performing practices allowing for child and practice characteristics

Position	Crude uptake (%)	Child population	Locational characteristics
1	96.7	31	Young professionals; commuter village
2	100.0	18	Mature professionals; suburb
3	85.2	54	Young professionals; suburb
4	60.2	65	Working class; mixed tenures; urban
5	81.7	60	Working class; inner city terraces
6	100.0	11	Older local authority estate
7	84.8	33	Mature professionals; suburb
8	79.0	43	Working class; mixed tenures; inner city
9	100.0	9	Mature professionals; suburb
10	96.7	31	Young professionals; mixed tenures; urban

Source: After Jones and Moon (1991).
N.B. 12 practices had crude uptake rates of 100%.

operating at different 'levels'. In the case of immunisation, the technique allows the researcher to separate out the effects of individual-level characteristics and characteristics relating to a higher level – neighbourhoods or surgeries. It is possible to assess the relative importance of each level and the variability within and between levels. The residual variation, remaining at the practice level after accounting for child and practice characteristics, known to be related to low uptake can be conceptualised as a 'contextualised performance indicator'. Jones and Moon compared performance on the problematic pertussis element of the immunisation uptake indicator using the multilevel approach and the traditional percentage uptake measure across 126 practices. On the crude measure, they found 12 practices reporting 100 per cent uptake, while 49 per cent of practices had uptake levels that would have contributed towards at least the lower level of target payment. Table 3.3 reveals those practices performing significantly better than average using the multilevel contextualised performance indicator. It shows clearly that good performance, given the nature of the practice and the client population, is possible with less than complete coverage of the target population.

The key conclusion from multilevel model work is that target payments fail to take account of the difficulties faced by some GPs and, in effect, favour those who need to make least effort, since, in some areas, a high uptake rate may be more easily achieved. One potential consequence would be a temptation to manipulate lists to exclude potential non-immunisers and thus minimise the threat to practice income that they pose. Leese and Bosanquet (1992) suggested that this shortcoming indicated a case for both special local development programmes in problem areas to improve recall systems and differential target setting for practices facing particular difficulties.

In the event, these cautionary notes stemming from work conducted at the time of the implementation of the 1990 contract have not been borne out. Even as early as 1992, Leese and Bosanquet were able to state that the introduction of target payments to GPs appeared to have had some effect in increasing uptake rates, particularly in some inner city areas. In the same year, the DoH (1992b) was able to indicate that the percentage of GPs receiving the higher-rate payment had increased from 56 per cent in the first year of the contract to 77 per cent in the second year, and the total percentage receiving target payments had risen over the same period from 81 to 90 per cent. Ritchie *et al.* (1992), examining changes in immunisation performance in 95 general practices in the Grampian region after the introduction of the 1990 contract, found that the number of practices achieving a 90 per cent rate rose from 69 (73 per cent) to 87 (93 per cent) 18 months after the introduction of the 1990 contract, and only one practice failed to meet lower target levels of 70 per cent for primary immunisation.

More recent data for the same area as that covered by the Jones and Moon work at the start of the 1990s reveals that, where once 49 per cent of practices had uptake levels that would have contributed towards at least the lower level of target payment, that figure is now 96.55 per cent, and just 245 children had not completed the full DTP immunisation course by the age of two. This might still be problematic if all incompletely immunised children were in the same area and the pattern of incomplete immunisation remained the same over a number of years; a non-immune reservoir of susceptible individuals would be built up providing there was little population mobility. There is little evidence, however, that this is the case, and it must be concluded that, despite its shortcomings, the programme of target payments for childhood immunisations was an effective and successful incentive.

Conclusion

This chapter has considered general practice in the mid- and late-1980s and laid particular stress on the developing emphasis on the health promotion role of GPs. It should be clear that, by the end of the 1980s, general practice was a substantially more 'managed' service than it had once been and the autonomy of GPs had been significantly curtailed, largely by tying their remuneration to capitation and performance, but also by developing the role of the FPC. This process should be understood as part of a governmental agenda that was to unfold more markedly in the early 1990s for the rest of the NHS. It was an agenda of control and regulation allied with the promotion of choice on the part of the patient and greater financial awareness on the part of general practice.

The change agenda was certainly not achieved without pain and opposition from general practice. While, as has been seen, some elements of the changes were well in tune with Royal College objectives for the development of a quality service (RCGP 1985), others were an overt threat to freedom, autonomy and income. Nor, as Smith and Armstrong (1989) argue, was there necessarily any great support from the public for the changes that were proposed. Indeed, they note interestingly that, in a listing of criteria of good health care in general practice, the three items least highly valued by the general public were health education, being able to change doctor easily, and well-decorated and convenient premises, all high-profile criteria in governmental policy. The change agenda of the 1980s did, however, create a general practice that was increasingly attuned to a public health role for patients on a list rather than a responsive service to those attending the surgery. General practice had also become financially aware of and used to, if not happy about, a much increased regulatory burden. These qualities were to be important underpinnings of the subsequent fortunes of general practice in the reformed NHS of the 1990s.

4

Gatekeeping and Beyond – GP Fundholding and Commissioning Models

The functional relationship between general practice and hospital services was carved from intraprofessional demarcations in the years leading up to the creation of the NHS. While in many ways institutionalising professional arrangements, the system fortuitously reflected and pre-dated what has become a desirable characteristic in health care: a strong primary care tier that controls referrals to more expensive hospital care. Governments, however, paid little further attention to the gatekeeping function of primary care and, even when interest in general practice blossomed again in the 1980s, it was primarily directed towards controlling the rise in prescribing costs and, more tentatively, improving the quality of provision. The notion of encouraging GPs to become more discriminating in referral, or of incorporating GPs in service-planning, had not been given serious consideration.

Two decades later, the role of GPs has changed both substantially and irrevocably. Most obviously, GP fundholding catapulted some GPs into positions of power, and all GPs benefited vicariously from the newly focused attention of trusts and health authorities. The original attraction of fundholding for the government may have been its potential to enliven the internal market, but the limitations of fragmented, 'demand-response' purchasing became evident, and concerns about strategic direction emerged. The need to involve all GPs in strategic decision-making resulted in a number of approaches and, most significantly, the parallel development of locality commissioning models. In effect, the Labour government has built upon this approach in its separate proposals for health services in England, Wales and Scotland.

As this chapter will show, the justification for fundholding can only be partly explained by a recourse to basic economic theory whereby markets, even managed markets, operate more effectively when there is an adequate number of purchasers as well as providers. The government's admonishment to health authorities to solicit the views of all GPs, and its tacit support of locality commissioning in the presence of the relatively dispersed leverage of fundholders, was indicative of a broader rationale. The primary care-led approach endorsed by government (NHSE 1994a) has several important elements. It seeks to make hospital and other secondary services more cost-effective as well as more responsive to service users through an exposure to the critical appraisal of 'informed consumers'. GPs, by virtue of their medical expertise and their proximity to service users, are held to be supremely placed to carry out this function. Implicit in this approach is the assumption that some services will be relocated within the primary care sector, provided that such change can be proved to be cost-effective. These attributes, it is assumed, would both exploit and enhance the benefits of a strong primary care infrastructure, described by Starfield (1997:687) as:

> the achievement of equity, effectiveness and efficiency by virtue of its defining characteristics: first contact access, longitudinality of practitioner–patient relationships, comprehensiveness of services available and provided to meet all but the least common needs of the population.

Not only GP fundholding, but also locality commissioning, and more recently primary care groups (PCGs) in England (Local Health Groups [LHGs] in Wales) are intrinsic to the development of the health service's – or *services'* – primary care-led approach. In Scotland, there will be some devolution of commissioning functions, but the Health Boards retain much broader responsibilities than those of their counterparts in England and Wales. This chapter will explore the rationale for and chart the progress of GP-focused initiatives in commissioning services, from the radical experiment of fundholding and more localised responses, to the Labour government's proposals for more collaboratively pitched arrangements. While it is recognised that both fundholding and the recent reforms offer the potential for GPs to address inefficiencies within and also performance variations between primary care practices, these aspects will be dealt with superficially here (see Chapters 3 and 5 for a further discussion of this area). Instead, this chapter will focus on locality commissioning initiatives and the role of fundholding in its various forms. In doing so, it will attempt to evaluate their success in relation to securing more efficient, responsive and equitable services.

GP Fundholding – Genesis and Catalysis

While the proposal in *Working for Patients* (DoH 1989a) to sever the umbilical cord between hospitals and community services and district health authorities was considered a dramatic enough proposal for some, the most radical of all was the opportunity for some GPs to become fundholders. The evolution of *Working for Patients* is well documented (see Butler 1992, Klein 1995, Timmins 1995). After abandoning any serious reconsideration of the funding of the NHS, the review group determined that greater efficiency could be squeezed from the system by ending the certainties surrounding the funding of individual hospitals and community services. Instead, the White Paper encouraged them to secure contracts from 'purchasers' in a climate of threatened, if not actual, competition. Further details of the proposals are provided in Table 4.1, and accounts of the internal market can be found in Klein (1995), Ranade (1997), Øvretveit (1995) and Baggott (1994). The idea of GP fundholding, first mooted by Maynard (1986), was a further flourish to the basic plan to fissure the tiered bureaucracy of the NHS along a purchaser–provider divide. The rationale for fundholding was that it would greatly enhance the number of purchasers, thereby encouraging a more vigorous internal or quasi-market, and that it would create a category of purchasers who were closest to the true consumers of health care – patients.

The idea was loosely based on the concept of HMOs in the USA. These have an enrolled population for whom they undertake to provide primary and secondary health care for an annual sum, although HMO plans often require patient co-payments for treatments. Such arrangements, which place the financial risks of mismanagement at the door of HMOs, contrast with fee-

Table 4.1   The basics of the internal market

● District health authorities (DHAs) as purchasers delegated responsibility for service provision to hospital and community trusts (providers). DHAs responsible for monitoring provision against a number of performance indicators

● DHAs commissioned health care for patients of non-fundholding GPs and an extensive range of services for patients of fundholders. Potential providers included hospital and community trusts, the commercial and voluntary sectors

● GP fundholders were permitted to manage their own budgets and were able to purchase a limited but growing menu of investigations, treatments and services from hospital and community trusts and other, non-NHS providers

● Family Practitioner Services (FPSs)/Family Health Service Authorities (FHSAs) assumed additional responsibilities for monitoring GP services, prescribing and budgets. FHSAs were merged with DHAs to form health authorities in 1996

● Trusts were given more freedom to develop their services, buy and sell assets, and set pay and conditions. Capital charges were laid against their assets in order to create a 'level playing field' with non-NHS competitors

● Resource management was introduced to all trusts. Hospital doctors were required to take part in medical audit. General managers became involved in the allocation of merit awards for consultants

● The remit of the Audit Commission was extended to include the NHS

---

for-service systems that have been implicated in rising health care costs in the USA and elsewhere. HMO physicians, whether they profit-share or, as employees, work within performance-related pay systems, have an incentive to control the costs of care. Standards of care are presumed to be maintained by a competitive market and ultimately by the threat of litigation. The concept of fundholding, although partly modelled on that of the HMO, had to be grafted onto a health care system relatively uninitiated in the practice of managed care and with units (GP practices) with much smaller enrolled populations than occur in HMOs. There were therefore risks inherent in the impact of catastrophic costs of the statistically unpredictable on comparatively small budgets (such as the once-in-a-GP-lifetime heart transplant case) or those associated with possible maladroit management.

Accordingly, GP fundholding began cautiously, the government restricting the scheme to group practices with a minimum threshold of 11,000. These were able to purchase a limited menu of the commonplace and less costly investigations and procedures. Subsequently, the threshold was progressively lowered to 5,000 and the range of purchasable procedures and services was extended. In 1994, two additional categories of fundholding were created. Community fundholding enabled the more wary practices to hold funds for community nursing services and prescribing, while, at the other end of the spectrum, total fundholding pilot schemes, also known as total purchasing pilots (TPPs) were constituted to meet or approximate the full range of commissioning requirements for a substantial population. In addition to such 'top-down' initiatives, some fundholders responded to local market conditions by creating multifunds. These, as the name suggests, pooled funds to gain more leverage on providers and reduce administrative costs via economies of scale. The problem for such large structures would be the maintenance of an 'ecological' approach to commissioning, remaining sensitive to those needs articulated by patients as well as those estimated from epidemiological and other research-based data.

The government in essence eliminated financial risks to GPs and reduced the potential problem of adverse selection (whereby fundholders preferentially register the fitter categories of patient on their lists) by defining the purchasing allowance as a fund rather than a budget. If fund overspends were not subsequently corrected by improved financial management, GPs risked losing their status as fundholders but nothing worse. Funds also included indicative prescribing costs and an allowance for staffing costs. Fundholders were allowed to vire funds between these areas and to reinvest end-of-financial-year underspends on initiatives that benefited patient care. These arrangements, together with additional management allowances and, not infrequently, health authority investments in practice-based information technologies, made fundholding an attractive prospect for some. In the first wave in April 1991, approximately 7 per cent of GPs in England became fundholders, and by 1996 the symbolically important target of 50 per cent of fund-holding GPs, covering 51 per cent of the population in England, was achieved (NHSE 1997). By the end of 1996 in Wales, 39 per cent of the population were covered by fundholding practices (Welsh Office 1998a). In contrast, fund-holding never got under way in Scotland, achieving a coverage of less than 20 per cent of the population (Groves 1999).

The balance sheet for fundholding is somewhat complicated. One of the ambitions of the scheme was that it would secure improvements in service quality and efficiency. Glennerster *et al.* (1994) carried out an early study covering the first three waves of fundholder in three regions. Noting that the expression of fundholders' purchasing power related to particular hospital services that had not tended to perform well, they determined that fund-holders in their study had been able to secure improvements. In other words, the changes were reactive, driven by experience with the objective of meeting individual patients' needs – what Freeman (1996:62) calls 'bespoke purchasing' – as opposed to adopting a longer-term view of service development. The Audit Commission (1996) similarly found that the majority of fundholders whom they surveyed sought an improvement in the quality of services, including reduced waiting times, a wider choice for patients and better communication from hospitals.

So much for 'process' efficiency, but what of the efficiency of resource allocation within hospital services and between the secondary and primary care sectors? The results of studies are somewhat equivocal. Coulter and Bradlaw (1993) found no change in the level of referral patterns or change between primary and secondary care settings in their study of first-wave fundholders in an English regional health authority. This contrasts with the findings of a study based in Scotland (Howie *et al.* 1992), which showed a reduction in the number of referrals to secondary care facilities but an increase in the use of direct access services that do not require the sanction of a hospital consultant. A minority of fundholders in the Audit Commission's survey were also purchasing a higher than average number of day surgery procedures, a result that should be set against a steady rise in day case procedures overall.

Glennerster and colleagues (1994) offer a tentative but fitting conclusion in their study: that fundholding had been the catalyst of a more searching approach to resource allocation in health service-planning. Fundholding thus seems to have made some improvements in the efficiency of services and possibly in the allocation of resources between primary and secondary care sectors, but this seems largely to have been based on local or 'impressionistic' knowledge. This is, of itself, not necessarily problematic – one does not need research and audit to identify a poor service – but it is preferable that service developments should, wherever possible, be informed by evidence-based research. Disconcertingly, the Audit Commission observed that fundholders made limited use of the evidence of effectiveness.

TPPs, usually agglomerations of experienced fundholders anxious to extend the range of purchasing, were initially established for a period of three years (1995–98) but were overtaken, like other forms of fundholding, by the Labour government's decision to defer the eighth fundholding wave in 1997. There are some similarities between PCGs and TPPs, both of which bring a population focus to commissioning. Thus, the findings of a major programme of evaluative research, commissioned by the Department of Health (DoH), may be instructive for PCG development. Mays *et al.* (1998) found that the projects were selective in that they did not cover the full range of commissioning responsibilities undertaken by a health authority for a population. TPPs experienced difficulties in acquiring and handling adequate data on costs and activities and, like the standard fundholding practices from which they had evolved, did not formally assess patient needs when establishing purchasing objectives, using instead the personal knowledge of the GPs. Purchasing ambitions were modest and incremental in scope, concentrating on obvious problem areas, where there was the greatest likelihood of success (Mays *et al.* 1997).

One of the most serious concerns voiced in relation to fundholding was that it would create a less equitable service (Whitehead 1994, Coulter 1995, Mohan 1995). Indeed, it is hard to see how, if the objective of fundholding was to secure an improvement in services for practice patients, inequities could be prevented. There is certainly some evidence that fundholders' patients experienced shorter waiting times for elective procedures (Kammerling and Kinnear 1996, Dowling 1997), yet the Audit Commission found that two-thirds of those fundholders setting targets for reduced waiting times adopted their local health authority's standards, thus eliminating, in theory, the potential for inequity. The greater potential of fundholders to exploit the market nevertheless enabled some fundholders' patients to experience shorter waiting times in comparison with those for whom access had been negotiated by a health authority. This success probably relates to fundholders' threatened volatility as purchasers: they could more readily withdraw custom from a trust than could the 'bulk-purchasing' health authorities, and could exploit shorter waiting lists of more distant providers with one-off referrals. TPPs, if anything, could exert greater purchasing power over providers, but their impact on equity remains obscure since 'there was little [health authority] action to monitor equity between TPP and non-TPP populations' (Mays *et al.* 1998:vii). In contrast, non-fundholding GPs had little flexibility or leverage; they were required to refer patients to contracted providers or were forced to embark on negotiations with the health authority in order to secure an extracontractual referral.

However, the assumption that fundholding practices alone achieved improvements for their patients has to be treated with caution. With the exception of queue-jumping, many changes introduced into hospital services at the behest of fundholders are likely to have been implemented for all patients. This is particularly true for those areas in which health authorities worked closely with fundholders and non-fundholders to elicit strategic improvements in care (see, for example, Dawson 1996, Greagsby and Milner 1996), although such arrangements might have been exemplars rather than the rule. The Audit Commission (1996) commented on the lack of collaboration between health authorities and fundholders over strategic commissioning and the lack of articulation between health authority purchasing strategies and GPs generally. The consequences of this for successful implementation have been reported elsewhere (North 1997a, 1998). However, any assessment of the impact of fundholding on equity of outcomes is compromised by a dearth of research.

The evaluation of fundholding has thus been jeopardised by the absence of any systematic review by government and by the problem of isolating fundholding outcomes from more general developments in the NHS, such as the waiting list initiative. Further difficulties of assessment arise from the relatively short period of fundholding's existence, a factor that is even more germane to evaluations of TPPs. The full-blown internal market was in operation from 1992 onwards (after a year of steady state during which health authorities were proscribed with regard to changing commissioning arrangements) and effectively ceased in June 1997, when the New Labour government signalled the end of the experiment by discontinuing the eighth wave of fundholders. *The New NHS* confirmed the cessation of fundholding after April 1999, as did the proposals for Wales, Scotland and Northern Ireland. The replacements for fundholding, PCGs, and in Wales LHGs, are discussed later in this chapter, along with the rather different arrangements for Scotland, but, for the present, other forms of GP involvement in commissioning will first be reviewed.

GP Commissioning – a Diversity of Forms

'Mosaic' is the term aptly used by Smith *et al.* (1997) to describe the variety of approaches to primary care commissioning. The variety uncovered by these researchers and others (Meads 1996, BMA 1997) is a testament to the imagination and innovatory energy of both managers and GPs. In some instances, the configurations were purchaser reactions to local market conditions in that GP fundholders pooled resources to create more powerful purchasing partnerships, as well as to achieve economies of scale in management overheads. Elsewhere, the stimulus was the DoH's requirement that health authorities consult with local GPs to establish appropriate purchasing arrangements. The mosaic described by Smith and colleagues also included patches where GPs, for ideological reasons, refused any involvement in alternative approaches to commissioning.

Since fundholding initially covered only modest proportions of the population, and the menu of purchasable treatments and investigations was limited, the bulk of services were commissioned by health authorities. Moreover, if money were to follow patients, authorities had to find out where GPs would prefer to send their patients for care. In addition to this rudimentary assessment of patterns of demand, health authorities were required to consult GPs, along with others, on the development of priorities and new service models that would better meet the needs of the local population (NHSME 1991a, 1991b). The strategic role of health authorities, and specifically their partnership with GPs, was reinforced by the publication of *Towards a Primary Care-led NHS*, which stated that 'all GPs, whether fundholding or not, will be more involved in developing local health strategies' (NHSE 1994a:3). More pragmatically, if a health authority could offer non-fundholders an opportunity to exert influence without converting to fundholding, its future was also more secure.

It is not difficult to see why GPs, particularly fundholders, should be preeminent in commissioning. While health authorities had the resources and experience to predict the probable needs of local populations and to identify treatments and service models that offered the best outcomes for patients, fundholders increasingly held the balance in purchasing arrangements. This was not simply a matter of crude financial leverage, of fundholders contributing a significant tranche of provider income for specific services, although this was important. More fundamentally, it reflected the unwelcome political consequences of an absence of fundholders' support for a health authority's purchasing strategies. In addition, the frequent lack of convincing evidence in support of any one particular service model, or the sheer complexity of evidence to be weighed in decision-making, commended a consensual approach (North 1998). Thus, without the involvement of fundholders and non-fundholding GPs, the legitimisation of purchasing strategies and priorities would have proved extremely difficult.

Both the BMA survey (1997) and Smith *et al.*'s (1997) research are testimony to the complexity and dynamism of commissioning arrangements. The BMA identified three basic categories: centrally based advice, GPs being nominated members of a health authority's decision-making body for purchasing; group-based advice, in which a health authority solicited the opinion of groups not necessarily reflective of all local GP opinion; and locality-based advice from established GP groups for the purpose of commissioning. Fundholders were generally fully integrated into arrangements, about 40 per cent of health authorities indicating separate forums for fundholders to contribute to the commissioning process. The West Midlands study (Smith *et al.* 1997), in which fundholders constituted between 40 per cent and 85 per cent of health authorities' GP populations, found a diversity of models within as well as between health authorities, multifunds co-existing alongside GP commissioning groups. The authors, however, observed that a locality focus 'was of universal importance' (1997:30).

Balogh (1996) identifies the origins of locality planning in the early 1980s. The two projects she describes, based in Exeter and Pimlico, embraced an approach that attempted to mediate the views of local professional and community groups in service development. According to Balogh, these epitomised many aspects of the community health movement. The emphasis on participative, democratic processes and social action that is characteristic of the movement is not, however, pre-eminent in the more recent locality commissioning models, in which primary care, and in particular general practice, appear to have been the represented constituencies. The devolution and decentralisation of decision-making, which are, prima facie, assumed to deliver a more democratic process, have in the NHS been associated with a changed managerial culture and the internal market, and have been heavily influenced by medical opinion. The Conservative government's preference was for a consumerist model within which fundholding 'businesses' found early acclaim for their responsiveness and dynamism. Certainly, a large organisation cannot be run by plebiscite, and the complexity of health care requires informed and often finely balanced judgements, but while some decisions might undoubtedly be indicated by research-based evidence and rational, informed debate, others are more value laden or contentious. These are grounds for a more inclusive process, which locality models are well placed to generate. Whether or not locality commissioning was seen as a prelude to more pluralistic commissioning processes, these have, to some degree, attempted to build on pre-existing community identities.

Just as there have been differences between locality commissioning and other approaches to GP involvement in commissioning, so there are varied models of locality commissioning. As Hudson (1994) indicated, the degree of budgetary devolution varied within a range extending from a central purchasing model to totally devolved budgeting. In the central purchasing model, localities may simply have offered advice to the health authority/commission that contributed to authority-wide contracts or, in a stronger version, more locally specific contracts. Still more potent models of locality commissioning were defined by devolved budgets and locality-designated health authority managers. Localities were not exclusive to non-fundholders, and an important characteristic has been the proportion of fundholders in their membership. This is particularly the case where the GPs concerned have adopted a more collegiate approach to service development, since fundholders provided the financial clout that localities might otherwise have lacked.

Finally, there appeared to be differences in the degree to which localities involved other agencies and community representatives in their deliberations. A cursory examination of the literature reveals a wide range of processes, ranging from the non-apparent to the more evident but infrequent consultation exercise and the determinedly participative approach of one locality in the North East (Freake *et al.* 1997). It may well be that localities preferred to leave this task to health authorities. The NHS Management Executive (NHMSE) initiative *Local Voices* (1992a) required health authorities to consult with their local communities. Consultation using Community Health Councils (CHCs) and public meetings were the most favoured methods adopted by health authorities in the BMA (1997) survey, but Ham's (1992b) early study found that consultation initiatives were centred on localities. Accounts of several locality projects after 1992 suggested that they concentrated on involving GPs (Balogh 1996). Thus, the earlier, more pluralistic conceptualisation of 'locality' was less in evidence and may have required the sponsorship of local champions in order to thrive.

As with fundholding, there has been no systematic evaluation of locality commissioning by government, although a number of smaller studies have been undertaken by external researchers or local health service personnel (Balogh 1995, Freake *et al.* 1997, Hine and Bachmann 1997, Smith and Shapiro 1997, Smith *et al.* 1997). Several themes emerge from these studies. GPs commonly appreciated the improved communication between practices (Hine and Bachmann 1997) and the benefits of working more cooperatively, findings that belie the traditional view of GPs as robustly independent operators (Smith *et al.* 1997). However, Smith *et al.* also found that many GPs were concerned to preserve their independence and were wary of their incorporation into larger structures, a sentiment that, if generally felt by GPs, might not bode well for future GP-led commissioning in the UK. Hine and Bachmann reported improved communication with health authorities, a finding implicit in other studies, including the BMA's (1997) survey of commissioning activities. An engagement with other agencies, such as housing and social services, as well as with community groups, was also evident in some studies. Smith *et al.* (1997) reported closer working relationships with social services personnel at strategic and operational levels within some of the West Midlands projects in the study. Service user involvement was not widely reported within the locality- or practice-sensitive projects; where efforts were made, they tended to be restricted to patient satisfaction surveys. Evidence of a more committed approach to community involvement can be found in a Newcastle locality project, in which the conclusion was that a dialogue between general practice and the community had been established 'on a more equal basis' (Freake *et al.* 1997:29).

Processual outcomes such as these are important if locality commissioning and its successors are to work effectively, but the improvement of services at both primary and secondary levels is the litmus test of locality commissioning. Any evaluation of this is problematic since there are a limited number of published studies with detailed outcome evaluations. Nor is it possible to determine from the literature the impact, if any, of localities holding or not holding budgets. Positive outcomes were claimed, the more prominent of these being accounts of improvements in community-based services delivered by other providers, such as mental health services and outreach services or one-stop clinics. There was also evidence of the development of practice-based services such as physiotherapy, counselling and attached social workers. In addition, improvements in hospital-based services, for example the reduction of waiting lists for specific conditions, had been targeted (Willis 1996, Hine and Bachmann 1997, Smith and Shapiro 1997).

Some of the services targeted were similar to those described in evaluations of fundholding (Glennerster *et al.* 1994, Audit Commission 1996), even to the degree that investment had occurred in some services in which cost-effectiveness was difficult to determine. More positively, Willis reported administrative economies in two commissioning projects (East Dorset and Nottingham) that compared favourably with the costs of fundholding. This may well have been the case in other locality projects, but elsewhere there was evidence of concern over the investment of GP resources in locality commissioning and the need for appropriate support (Hine and Bachmann 1997, Smith and Shapiro 1997).

It is a futile exercise to compare locality commissioning with fundholding. Partly because of the range of models within each approach, significant differences can dissolve away depending on particular selections. For example, in terms of commissioning, how does a consortium of fundholders on the Isle of Wight differ from a locality in County Durham with a total devolution of resources? Moreover, the involvement of standard fundholders in locality purchasing not only drew them into commissioning activities, but also lent some of their positive attributes, such as their dynamism not to mention their financial leverage, to locality activities.

While the Conservative government was in power, localities were not seen as an alternative to fundholding, the presumption being that there would be a steady attrition of non-fundholding intransigents. Instead they provided a means of soliciting GPs' views on service-planning, a process qualitatively different from that of purchasing, and of reconciling the practice-based focus of fundholding with the more panoramic, population-focused gaze of localities. The Conservatives' preference, set out in *Primary Care: Delivering the Future* (DoH 1996a) was to give health authorities responsibility for bringing together primary care, secondary care and local authorities to develop locally agreed health care strategies (Section 2.20). This would have ensured that fundholding practices inevitably became involved in commissioning as opposed to simply purchasing. The proposals for pilot schemes submitted to the DoH as a consequence of *Delivering the Future* were, in the event, selected and commissioned by a Labour government determined to end fundholding but supportive of GPs' close involvement in health care commissioning. Within a few months, the concept was overtaken by proposals in Labour's White Papers for health services in England, Wales and Scotland.

Primary Care and Future Commissioning

Although in Scotland the health service reforms (Scottish Office Department of Health 1997) have seemingly been more conservative, *The New NHS* (DoH 1997) has expanded the role of England's GPs in commissioning services, as has the White Paper for Wales, *NHS Wales: Putting Patients First* (DoH/Welsh Office 1998) (Table 4.2). In Northern Ireland, proposals (DHSS 1998) to create Primary Care Cooperatives (similar to PCGs but with budgets for health and social care) have been delayed as a consequence of the failure to make progress towards a National Assembly; fundholding continues as an interim arrangement. Whether because of lack of progress or a certain degree of 'anglocentricity' in the media and academia at the time of writing, much of the commentary has focused on the reforms in England. The discussion that follows to some extent, is hostage to these limitations.

Dismissing the argument between fundholding and non-fundholding alternatives as 'yesterday's debate' (Section 5.6:33), *The New NHS* instead introduced PCGs. This is locality commissioning by any other name, but with the difference that resources for primary care are incorporated into PCG budgets. Embryonic PCGs were allowed some discretion in deciding at which stage they wished to enter, although the most evolved stage was proscribed in year 1; there was, however, an expectation that PCGs would progress through the stages. The White Paper for Wales appeared rather more equivocal about the devolution of commissioning responsibilities to LHGs. All began as health authority subcommittees (equivalent to stage 1 PCGs), further development being contingent on the demonstration of particular qualities, giving the impression that this would be the exception rather than the rule.

Scotland's blueprint was very different from that of either England or Wales. The rural composition of much of Scotland, with its consequent provider monopolies, had offered little incentive for fundholding. The lack of GP commissioning experience, coupled with the difficulties of collaboration imposed by geography, is a further explanation of the government's strategy, which preserved the commissioning function of the 15 Health Boards. More radically, Primary Care Trusts in Scotland (SPCTs) have, from the outset, been configured from both primary care and community health services. GPs are

Table 4.2 Health services reforms in England, Wales and Scotland

Country and name of commissioning organisation	Policy document	Board membership	Functions	Accountable to
England Primary Care Groups (PCGs)	*The New NHS: Modern, Dependable* (DoH 1997)	GP chair and majority membership; nurse, social work and lay representatives; executive officers	Stage 1: advisory Stages 2/3: service commissioning and development	Stages 1 and 2 : subcommittee to health authority with internal accountability Stage 3: free-standing body, accountable to health authority
Primary Care Trusts (PCTs): PCGs merged with part/all of community trusts		Unclear at time of writing	Management of primary and community services (including community hospitals in some areas) and commissioning of secondary (acute) care	Accountable to health authorities (or possibly mega-health authorities) for operational management of PCTs and strategic development of local health services

(cont'd)

Table 4.2 (cont'd)

Country and name of commissioning organisation	Policy document	Board membership	Functions	Accountable to
Wales Local Health Groups	*NHS Wales: Putting Patients First* (DoH/Welsh Office 1998)	As for PCGs	Subcommittees of health authorities initially, with indicative budgets for Hospital and Community Health Services (HCHS) prescribing and practice infrastructure	Internal accountability to one of five Welsh health authorities for devolved responsibilities
Scotland GPs members of Local Health Care Cooperatives (LHCCs). LHCCs are formally associated with Scottish primary care trusts (SPCTs), the latter incorporating primary care and community health services	*Designed to Care. Renewing the National Health Service in Scotland* (Scottish Office Department of Health 1997)	LHCCs are expected to play an integral role in the direction of primary care within SPCTs. SPCTs have the right to hold the budget for primary and community health services. Joint investment funds available for secondary care clinicians and GPs to develop clinical services	Strong lead by Health Boards, who will have overall steerage of service development and budgets for secondary care	SPCTs not given as extensive a range of commissioning responsibilities, as PCGs will potentially have, but accountable to Health Boards for devolved functions

expected to play a central role in directing and managing these new organisations via the voluntary grouping of GPs in Local Health Care Cooperatives (LHCCs). Health Boards will devolve budgets for primary and community care to SPCTs rather than LHCCs, so the degree to which GPs become involved in local commissioning is contingent on their participation in SPCTs.

SPCTs could therefore model some aspects of commissioning activities for PCGs in England, where there are four stages of PCG. The entry level, for those inexperienced or faint of heart, requires GPs (England) to act in an advisory capacity to health authorities, which, in effect, continue to commission services. Stages 2 and 3 devolve commissioning responsibilities to PCGs, which hold budgets for prescribing, secondary care and non-GMS costs (covering staff and other general medical services practice costs). These arrangements are similar to those for fundholding but, unlike the situation with fundholders, PCG overspends will not be bailed out by health authorities. PCGs also cover populations of around 100,000, whereas a standard fundholding practice of six partners would have a list size of, on average, approximately 12,000.

The agenda set for the NHS, and consequently for PCGs, is much broader than before (Table 4.3). Health authorities are charged with monitoring performance, surrendering much of their former, active role in the pursuit of NHS objectives by way of commissioning and the orchestration of fundholding activities. At stage 4, PCGs metamorphose to Primary Care Trusts (PCTs), which may incorporate community health services presently managed by community trusts. PCTs, the largest of which will be the UK's closest approximation of HMOs in the USA, will thus be responsible for providing or secondarily commissioning a large range of primary or ambulatory care services, as well as commissioning secondary care. If PCTs eventually merge or affiliate, they may take over responsibility for tertiary or specialised commissioning, thereby ending health authority commissioning responsibilities.

Although stages 2 and 3 give PCGs the ability to transfer resources from secondary to primary care, it is likely that PCTs will most potentiate this. As

Table. 4.3   The Labour Government's objectives for health and social care

- Reduce inequalities and improve the health of the population
- Encourage service integration where appropriate
- Boost standards by improving the quality and responsiveness of services
- Achieve better performance and efficiency
- Enable staff to optimise their contribution
- Improve public confidence in social services and the NHS

Source: NHSE 1998.

providers and managers of a larger range of facilities and health care employees, PCTs will have the capacity and incentive to introduce services that make maximum use of care in lower-dependency hospital units or in the community. This will not mean that decisions about the prioritisation of care will be any easier to make. The introduction of new technologies is likely to stimulate demand as much as reduce costs in both community or acute care settings, although the output of the National Institute for Clinical Excellence (NICE) and the National Service Frameworks will provide compelling guidance.

In contrast, SPCTs are not directly responsible for commissioning all services but form a triangular partnership with Health Boards and hospital trusts to plan services. In that SPCTs are expected to lead discussions on services at the interface of primary and secondary care, their role and that of the GP-led LHCCs is a potentially powerful one. There have, however, been reports of dissatisfaction among Scottish GPs over the absence of the GPs' pivotal control of the commissioning process, as in England (Hopton and Heaney 1999). These uncertainties are further compounded by the effect that devolution may have on future health care policy. Thus, for the present, it is difficult to speculate on the influence that Scotland's GPs will have on service development.

Whereas fundholding and locality commissioning appeared to have had only limited involvement with local authorities and community groups, the need for this was made explicit in *The New NHS* (DoH 1997). In the Scottish and Welsh White Papers, the health authorities and Health Boards appeared to retain more responsibility for interagency links, although in Wales the LHGs include voluntary organisation representation on their boards, offering the prospect of a more 'bottom-up' approach. Emphasising cooperation rather than competition, England's White Paper called for more collaborative working relationships between trusts and PCGs, as well as between health and social services. The governing bodies of PCGs/PCTs include community nursing and social services personnel, and PCGs are expected to demonstrate clear arrangements for public involvement. This may come as something of a culture shock for some GPs accustomed to acting with a degree of autonomy in the relative isolation of their practices, but involvement with other stake-holders in health and community care may be reserved for the few GPs who emerge as leaders of PCGs/PCTs.

Despite the idealism of *The New NHS* (DoH 1997), the arrangements for governing PCGs/PCTs are not especially democratic. The original tenor of the guidelines – that local processes for the development of PCGs should be inclusive of all stakeholders (HSC 1998/065 Section 12, NHS Executive) – was somewhat overwhelmed by concessions won by a powerful BMA lobby. Since GP practices were viewed by the government as being the 'basic building blocks of PCGs' (Milburn, quoted by Andalo 1998), GP support was seen as pivotal; consequently, they were accorded majority representation on and the chairpersonship of PCGs. The compromise arrangements delivered the GPs and ensured that the initiative would at least be launched, but, in subduing the original pluralistic inflections of the proposals, they may have unwittingly retarded effective interagency collaboration, as well as the development of formal and informal links with the community.

The 'embedding' of PCGs – and those LHGs that may evolve to enjoy greater responsibilities – in their local communities is essential if they are to gain legitimacy for some difficult decisions that will inevitably come their way as commissioners of health care. As non-budget-holders, most GPs were not held accountable for decisions on treatment priorities. Fundholding practices were absolved from the responsibility for funding treatments over a modest cost threshold. In contrast, PCGs from stage 2 onwards assume responsibility for resource allocation and, with it, the risk of the public's opprobrium if they do not carry them with them in debates about the prioritisation of services. GPs are aware of this. Research conducted in the first three months following the publication of the White Paper revealed that many GPs were concerned that PCG resources for commissioning would be inadequate and that the rationale for the reforms was essentially to make GPs responsible for rationing health care. While GPs were somewhat concerned with the representativeness of consultations with the broader community, they readily recognised the importance of a dialogue concerning commissioning priorities (North *et al.* 1999).

There are few apparent solutions. The record of patient consultation and/or participation in practices has not been impressive (see Chapter 8), nor has there been the perceived need or opportunity for initiatives focusing on wider communities. CHCs, which have historically monitored service provision, are not an obvious answer. Not only do they lack co-terminosity with localities, but it would also be difficult to find a compromise between a participatory function within PCGs and CHCs' traditional involvement in the prosecution of patients' complaints within the health service. Citizens' juries or health panels may be an option, but whatever approach to local consultation PCGs adopt, they must avoid tokenistic gestures and a commonplace and serious flaw in previous healthcare commissioning: a lack of clarity concerning the purpose of public involvement, which has served to exacerbate problems of the specific approach to be pursued (Lupton *et al.* 1998).

PCGs, and in Wales LHGs, offer the promise of strategic commissioning centred on a population's needs, a goal that was never entirely achievable with the more fragmentary approach of standard fundholding. Total fundholding came closest to this, but fundholding remained focused on a relatively narrow range of health services. Commissioning efficient services that improve the health of the community, reduce inequalities and interlock with social care services adds up to a complex agenda, albeit one that moves much closer to the WHO ideal for primary care identified at Alma Alta. The importance of collaboration with other statutory authorities and community groups in order to achieve this is recognised in the White Paper, but how the process will work in PCGs and LHGs is as yet uncertain. Effective joint planning between health authorities and social services has previously proved elusive (Audit Commission 1986, Griffiths 1988, Wistow 1995), and although this objective is central in the discussion document *Partnerships in Action* (DoH 1998a), its identification of a role for PCGs stages 1–3 is peculiarly circumspect. These issues are discussed further in Chapter 9.

GPs have in the past resolutely guarded their independence. They choose to work in small units where they operate relatively autonomously and, as employers, exercise control over others. Even within the primary health care team, which incorporates attached staff, GPs are often seen as team leaders. Practice-level dynamics such as these are, however, not appropriate for the more corporate, consensus-seeking style implicit in PCG governance. More positively, work arrangements in the form of shared on-call duties with other practices, and more recently the development of larger GP cooperatives, have extended the formal links between practices. Such functional arrangements enhance GP cooperation where collegiate relationships with medical colleagues are already the norm, but these may yet be put to the test in PCGs. GPs in one study (North *et al.* 1999) described their profession as having individualistic operating styles and furthermore predicted that any difficulties in reaching agreement would be compounded by the large number involved in PCGs (approximately 50–60 for an average-size PCG constituency).

There are, in addition, other potential stressors. PCG budgets cover prescribing costs, staffing costs and the use of secondary care (referral costs), and will inevitably involve the monitoring of individual practice performance in these areas. Outlier practices, which overspend on referrals or prescribing, may therefore become a source of friction between PCG members, and this may in turn contaminate other commissioning activities. The effectiveness of PCGs, which are likely to rely on consensus decisions, may thus be compromised. In Scotland, where the GP LHCCs exist to prescribe and to provide services within identified levels of resources, arrangements appear to have been negotiated locally. In Lothian, for example, the SPCT rather than LHCCs will carry the risk of non-member practices' prescribing budgets (personal communication, Hopton 1999).

Concluding Thoughts: Gatekeepers with Calculators

In the 10 years since *Working for Patients* (DoH 1989a) announced fund-holding, the role of GPs in the NHS has changed dramatically. As the first point of contact for the patient, they have traditionally controlled access to more expensive hospital-based care. Before fundholding, however, decisions were made solely on the basis of a clinical definition of need. Fundholders, although generally cushioned in the early years of the internal market by generous funds, were the first to experience the necessary association between needs and treatment costs, as well as the need to indulge in primitive forms of resource allocation, most notably between prescribing and other budgets in the funding package. There has been little systematic evaluation of fundholding, particularly in relation to patient outcomes, and even less on the more inclusive but less economically powerful locality commissioning models. However, the various models of GP incorporation into service development generated by the internal market in health care will no doubt come to be regarded as rudimentary evolutionary forms. The next stage in the development of the gatekeeper's role, that envisaged in stage 3 and 4 PCGs and possible future manifestations of LHGs, will require that all GPs adopt more efficient referral practices and, with others, help to develop local services. In association with this task, they will assume responsibility for decisions that allocate resources between as well as within health care programmes. Operating within fixed budgets, they will be expected to meet the needs of the local population and to optimise provision by the redistribution of resources. The way in which GPs manage patients will be increasingly defined throughout the UK by centrally framed treatment protocols covering primary as well as secondary care. It is a gatekeeper's role that bears little comparison with that of a decade ago and one that will have far-reaching consequences for the way in which GPs practise medicine.

5

Accounting for their Actions – Regulation and the GP

> The National Health Service in Britain could not ensure that doctors... would choose overnight to be 'better' doctors; all it could do was to provide that particular framework of social resources within which potentially 'better' medicine might be more easily chosen and practised. (Titmuss 1963:171)

Much has changed since Titmuss wrote these words. An increasing interest in what GPs do and how well they do it is a barometer not only of the increased importance of primary health care's role in the NHS, but also of the state's growing interest in regulating the performance of doctors and strengthening their accountability to government and to society. It is a process not restricted to the UK alone but one that reflects increasing international concern with the rising costs of health care. Economic imperatives, however, are not the only rationale for enhanced regulation. The trend also reflects a more mature public perception of the fallibility of medicine, which in the UK has recently been fuelled by dramatic and tragic events. It is also possible to locate explanations for the increase in regulation in the redefinition of the state's role and the encouragement of greater pluralism in welfare. The privatisation of welfare provision has left the NHS relatively unscathed, but it has not been isolated from moves to reinforce regulatory controls – the 'steering' rather than 'rowing' state. These explanations and the broad strategies visited on the NHS will be discussed in this chapter, but of particular interest will be those measures directly influencing general practice.

Accountability is concerned with holding individuals responsible for their actions by requiring them to explain or answer for these actions. As Day and Klein (1987) indicate, it is one dynamic within broader regulatory frameworks that establishes the operational conduct of organisations or individuals in society. In order to hold someone accountable, there must be recognisable standards by which delegated actions can be judged. These may be more readily appraised in some spheres of activity than in others, and they vary in their degree of explicitness. For example, they may exist as unequivocal performance objectives, as loosely defined organisational goals, such as making service provision more equitable, or as codes of behaviour that permit interpretation. To be accountable for one's actions or the actions of others requires that one has control over them; hence society does not hold those unable to discriminate between right and wrong for reasons of mental illness accountable for an illegal act, but may hold agencies and/or individuals accountable for a lack of duty of care that permitted the transgression in the first instance (Day and Klein 1987).

Day and Klein suggest that the current usage of the term 'accountability' is ambiguous and seek to distinguish between political accountability, in which those with delegated authority are answerable to the people, and managerial accountability, which is concerned with 'making those with delegated authority answerable for carrying out agreed tasks according to agreed criteria of performance' (1987:27). To these can be added a third category: professional accountability. In 1858 the state, in establishing the General Council of Medical Education and Registration (renamed the General Medical Council [GMC] in 1951), recognised the right of the medical profession to control the registration of doctors and police their conduct thereafter. In this model, the doctor undertakes to act in the interest of the patient; only peers are judged to be competent to undertake the complex assessment of her or his medical performance. Excepting those actions which resulted in criminal or civil proceedings in the courts – even judicial appraisal being circumscribed by the dependence of the process on expert medical witnesses – this essentially gave the profession a monopoly over the process, including the criteria by which performance was judged. Doctors have traditionally been accountable for their day-to-day clinical performance to professional colleagues, a process attenuated by the concept of clinical autonomy and the reluctance of colleagues to whistleblow. Furthermore, it is necessarily framed by the doctor's duty to do her or his best for the *individual* patient rather than a concern for the stewardship of scarce resources.

As well as delegating responsibility for self-regulation, in 1948 the state delegated power to doctors to run the NHS. The state's near-monopoly over health care provision allowed it considerable dominion over the global resources devoted to health care but surrendered control of the allocation of resources to doctors (Klein 1990). This was realised not so much in the organisational arrangements of the hospital sector, which did indeed legitimise and reflect medical interests, as in the degree of clinical autonomy that doctors enjoyed in their practice without concern for the opportunity costs of decisions, and not infrequently with a limited knowledge of treatment efficacy. The independent contractor status of GPs isolated them from the mainstream administration of the NHS. Thus, they had little opportunity to influence the health service in general, but these arrangements left them in control over what were, in effect, their own businesses.

General practice was administered somewhat effetely by Executive Committees and later by FPCs, on which GPs enjoyed representation. The jurisdiction of the Executive Committees (subsequently FPCs) was limited but covered, as health authorities still do, complaints about the failure of GPs to observe the terms of their contract. Nevertheless, the FPCs lacked the administrative muscle to monitor GP performance, and the GPs' independent contractor status, in particular its 'legal, financial, and psychological complexities' (Huntingdon 1993:34), undoubtedly discouraged a more robust style of management. A more fundamental explanation was that the need for closer surveillance had not yet emerged on the political agenda, but with the Conservatives' election to office in 1979, the days of relatively unrestrained managerial as well as clinical independence were numbered for GPs, as well as for their colleagues in the hospital sector.

Progenitors of Change

Several processes underpin the search for greater accountability in the NHS, some of which are germane to other public sector services in the UK and others of which are synchronous with international trends that seek to bring greater direction to medical practice. This has in part been the product of the critique of the medical profession that challenged the characterisation of the profession as altruistic, instead arguing that what distinguished it and other professions from 'occupations' was monopoly power (Freidson 1970a, 1970b) and its use to secure privilege, status and income (Johnson 1972, Larson 1977). Other critiques contradicted the role of medicine in improving the overall health of populations (McKeown 1979) or criticised the overmedicalisation of society (Illich 1976). The exposure of medicine to criticism from academia occurred at a time when consumerist groups were beginning to promote the patient's perspective of health care experiences.

The 1960s and 70s also saw the advancement of neo-liberalist theories that regarded state bureaucracies as unwieldy, profligate, insensitive to the needs of service users and unresponsive to the policy objectives of governments. Rational choice theory argued that it was impossible to operate a satisfactory social (collective) welfare function; individuals should therefore be enabled to make choices – and pay for them. The analysis also directed blame towards those in charge, who in the case of the NHS were the doctors, for promoting unnecessary increases in the scale of operations in order to secure greater prestige and security (Niskanen 1971). This was an argument that resonated with the sociological critiques of the professions as self-serving. In the UK, the Fabian-inspired confidence concerning what could be achieved by the welfare state and its professionals waned amidst growing concerns over its cost and the ability of, as well as the need for, the state to maintain it.

In comparison with that of the USA and other European states, UK health care has displayed a modest rate of expenditure growth, attention having centred more on improving productivity than on cost containment. Elsewhere, where central budgetary control does not exist, the burgeoning costs of health care have resulted in third-party payers (governments and/or insurers) redefining patient eligibility, increasing competitiveness within the health sector and bringing pressure to bear on practitioners. Whether the aim in public as well as in privatised health care systems has been to stabilise or reduce expenditure, improving cost-effectiveness has been an important component. Organisational restructuring has been a favoured strategy, either generated by market pressures or, in the case of socialised health care systems such as the NHS, orchestrated by government policy. Directly influencing the practice of practitioners perhaps offers greater potential in the UK, where equity of provision remains a notional political goal. Doubts over the clinical effectiveness of some medical care, coupled with variations in practice (Harrison and Pollitt 1994), have led to efforts to coordinate professional practice more effectively in order to deliver 'value for money'. What Pereira Gray *et al.* predicted – 'If in the future general practice is to retain its share of NHS resources, let alone increase that share, we may expect a demand for much more explicit evidence about value for money' (1986:1314) – has come to pass.

However, in comparison with the battery of regulatory controls available to US health care administrators, progress in the UK has been more limited. Moreover, clinical effectiveness is an inadequate substitute for cost-effectiveness (Maynard 1997), implicit in which is an acknowledgement of the preferencing of population-wide needs over those of the individual. The system of professional accountability, buffered as it has been by the concept of clinical autonomy, has not been sufficient to secure consistent and satisfactory clinical practice on the part of some doctors. Measures announced in *The New NHS* (DoH 1997) and subsequent guidance, *A First Class Service* (DoH 1998b), are likely to remove some of the ambiguities concerning good practice and open up the scrutiny of clinical performance to a wider audience – both essential preconditions for improved accountability.

There are other elements of performance for which a practitioner in the NHS could be held to account and which have been problematic. Citing other research, Pereira Gray *et al.* (1986) listed some examples of failed standards in general practice in the 1980s. In addition to variations in prescribing and referral practices, these included the fact that 20 per cent of the child population had not been immunised against polio, diphtheria and tetanus, the difficulties faced in some areas by the public in registering with a GP, inadequate patient records and, in some single-handed practices, a somewhat cavalier attitude towards answering the telephone. This account implicitly recognises that the accountability of doctors is not restricted to their individual clinical performance, but includes the management of the patient as a whole and, depending on the circumstances, may incorporate responsibility for the organisation of a general practice or hospital department. Additionally, GPs in England will, as members of PCGs, be held to account for resource allocation between services and client groups at the local level.

Whatever the difficulties in determining an acceptable standard for clinical activities, the criteria for evaluating managerial performance and the quality of difficult decisions are less robust, as is the power to take remedial action. The BMA has negotiated majority representation for GPs on the PCG boards in the certain knowledge that PCGs cannot operate without the GPs' support. Especially if their evidence is based on qualitative judgements, health authorities will find it difficult to take corrective action against PCG boards without the support of the GP constituency.

The search for measures that would demonstrate satisfactory performance and reassure society has also come from within the medical profession. In discussing practice guidelines as a mechanism for ensuring greater accountability, Klazinga (1994) identified the need of the medical profession to meet society's expectations of accountability amidst some failure of confidence. Following the evident failure of self-regulatory processes at the Bristol Royal Infirmary,[1] there is apparently a more urgent search for regulatory systems that will placate both government and the public. The damage may, however, have been done. As a *British Medical Journal* editorial noted, the trust that patients place in their doctors 'will never be the same again' (Smith 1998:1918). The government inquiry following the Bristol incident may well make recommendations that will fracture the profession's near-monopoly regulation of clinical performance.

While matters concerning clinical performance have been regarded as the proper concern of the profession, doctors have been less interested in resource management or in being held to account for the use of resources. As noted above, to be concerned about the cost of treatment was seen as threatening the doctor's duty of care to the individual patient. This formed an important part of the rationale of the BMA's early opposition to fundholding, as well as figuring in the decisions of individual GPs not to become fundholders (Robinson and Hayter 1995). Health care has, however, moved on regardless. The economic necessity of harnessing clinical decision-making, combined with the increasing significance of a public health approach to health care, has emphasised population rather than individual health care strategies. The promotion of primary health care, with its low-tech, clinical generalists, and which in the UK conveniently covers geographically organised populations, can be regarded as an obvious strategic response (Klein 1986, Royal College of General Practitioners 1996).

The above constellation of factors has thus resulted in a greater concern for what doctors, in particular GPs, do or do not do in relation to several levels of activity. These are: clinical performance (safe and effective treatment); the cost-effective management of the individual patient; contractual professional duties; the practice- or directorate-level management of services; and, increasingly, allocative decisions between services or client groups. Making doctors accountable in these differing domains of their professional activities may be achieved through different, but overlapping, models of accountability. As well as the professional, managerial and political models, Emanuel and Emanuel (1996) identify an economic model. The significance of this in the UK, which asserted the discipline of the market and the power to make providers accountable through the threat of exit, has waned. Instead *The New NHS* (DoH 1997) emphasises collaboration rather than competition. The various models of accountability and the domains of medical activity they affect will now be discussed in relation to GPs. In order to contextualise developments in general practice within the wider NHS, reference will also be made to strategies applied to doctors in secondary care.

Regulation and Accountability – the Professional Model

The medical profession's responsibilities in respect of self-regulation have incorporated both statutory and self-sponsored duties. The GMC has the clearest role in that it has the power to admit to and suspend doctors from the register. The Royal Colleges, while promoting the interests of their members, as academic organisations play a significant part in improving the quality of practice. There is a wide encouragement of peer review and audit of practice. As Harrison and Pollitt (1994) note, there have been a number of audit initiatives, both local and national, generated by the profession rather than by state or management. Four regular national audits, the first established in 1951, have examined maternal deaths, deaths following surgery, stillbirths and deaths in infancy, and suicides and homicides by people with mental illness. Both local and national initiatives were controlled by the profession and were confidential, involvement being voluntary, but *Working for Patients* (DoH 1990) invited both hospital clinicians and GPs to participate in local audits, arrangements for which were to be agreed between the profession and management. What emerged from negotiations between Whitehall and the profession was a system in which managers were to be allowed access only to aggregated data, individual clinicians were not to be identified in reviews, and there were to be no measures to discipline non-participants. An opportunity to strengthen external accountability had foundered.

While there has undoubtedly been a genuine desire, led by the Royal Colleges, to improve clinicians' standards of performance, the profession's interest in clinical audit following *Working for Patients* has seemed more like a pre-emptive strategy, aimed at securing control of the process by the profession before external agencies could do so. Both ambitions are, of course, compatible. Promoting the standards of the profession is perhaps an especially important objective of the youngest of the Royal Colleges, the Royal College of General Practitioners (RCGP), which has fought to establish general practice as an academic subdiscipline of the profession (see Chapter 2). Its endeavours include the development of clinical guidelines, which will presumably need to articulate with the output of NICE, and it plays an active role in reviewing standards and revalidating training practices. The Royal Colleges are not only responsible for the dissemination of good practice, but have in the past also initiated enquiries into practice standards (Hughes *et al.* 1997). Perhaps more forward-looking than other Royal Colleges, the RCGP has raised the issue of practitioner revalidation with its membership, a debate that has spread to the GMC. A pilot scheme for the revalidation of GPs was introduced in the autumn of 1999 (Pringle 1999), which may eventually become the model for the remainder of the profession.

Ultimately, the GMC remains the body to which individual members of the profession are accountable for their actions. Cases may be brought before the GMC as a result of court cases, as a result of complaints by patients, or because of complaints or referrals by colleagues or health authorities. The GMC was primarily concerned with hearing complaints for misconduct, but from July 1997, procedures were established to hear cases of deficient performance too. In addition, in something of a volte-face since an earlier admonition discouraged publicly stated views of others' performances,[2] it has placed an ethical responsibility on doctors to report inadequately performing colleagues (GMC 1998). This much broader catalogue of culpable transgressions makes the GMC's purview more congruous with society's concerns. As Klein (1998:153) observes: 'Competence rather than chastity... has become the touchstone of good medical practice.'

The Commission for Health Improvement, which is charged with monitoring standards of clinical performance in NHS trusts, including PCTs, is also required to refer individual clinicians to the GMC if their performance is found lacking. The new arrangements, particularly if they do bring about a change of culture in a hitherto entrenchedly defensive profession, are potentially very powerful. At the very least, they encourage a climate of opinion in which greater openness and more rigorous standards of self-appraisal obtain. For the present, the impact of these changes is difficult to discern. The number of doctors reported to the GMC's Preliminary Proceeding Committee in 1997 for inadequacies in relation to the treatment of patients was 106, of which 43 cases were forwarded to the Professional Conduct Committee

(PCC). The records do not discriminate between other doctors and GPs other than in the subcategory of 'inadequate or inappropriate treatment', in which 14 GPs' cases were presented to the PCC, in contrast with those of four hospital doctors (personal communication, GMC 1993). Future statistics, which will reflect the changes over a 12-month period and possibly a stronger disposition of the profession and public to use the system, may well demonstrate an upward and not altogether unhealthy trend.

Although laypersons sit on the PCC, the profession has established the standards of clinical performance by which cases are assessed. The insularity of this process may well change if proposals fleshing out details of *The New NHS* (DoH 1997) come to fruition. Standards of clinical performance in the NHS will be increasingly framed by the work of the NICE, whose membership is drawn not only from members of the health professions, but also from academics, health economists and those representing patients' interests (DoH 1997:Section 7.11–12). This could broaden discourses on what is or is not acceptable clinical performance and may become the primary agency in establishing standards of clinical performance against which members of the profession are assessed.

The GMC may be the final arbiter of the most serious cases of professional misconduct, but the model of professional accountability is essentially collegiate and in theory operates throughout the ranks of the profession. There are, however, strong indications that the implicit agreement between the state and the medical profession, by which the latter was allowed to self-regulate, is under threat. In its consultation document on clinical governance in the NHS, the Blair government has nailed its colours to the mast, declaring that 'The organisation of professional self-regulation still owes more to history than to the need of patients in a modern NHS' (DoH 1998a:Section 3.46). Although in the future the contribution of the profession in establishing appropriate standards of clinical practice will remain paramount, what is likely to change is the range of strategies employed to evaluate performance, extending the scope of evaluation beyond the narrow criterion of clinical competence. Similarly, the locus of regulatory authority will increasingly reside with the state rather than the profession.

The Managerial Model

Earlier discussions noted the growing significance of the state's role in managing medical activities and holding practitioners directly to account, rather than through delegated authority to the medical profession. It is a proactive process that seeks to mould medical activities in particular ways, which respond to the perceived needs of the health service as defined by government rather than to the profession's preferences. One of the more obvious strategies for strengthening the accountability of hospital doctors for resource management was to incorporate them within the management structure of the NHS. Recognising the failure of consensus decision-making, Griffiths proposed a more robust managerial system that tied performance objectives to localised budgets and encouraged doctors to become closely involved in the day-to-day management of resources (DHSS 1983). Many doctors, however, eschewed incorporation as managers in the reorganised NHS and were suspicious of the new breed of manager (Strong and Robinson 1990, Pollitt *et al.* 1991). Critically, doctors were not accountable to managers for the effective management of resources; the levers to achieve this were not available until the 1990 reorganisation and the introduction of competition, albeit more perceived than real, to the NHS.

Managerial control was slow to come to general practice. The indictment of FPCs as being somewhat ineffective organisations is attributable not so much to the fragmented nature of general practice or to the strong presence of GP members on the Committees, as to the impotence of the original contract struck with the profession. The government could make some of the more ineffective and therefore costly clinical decisions out of bounds, as it indeed achieved with the limited list of prescribed drugs introduced in 1985 in order to reduce the accelerating costs of prescribing. However, even this rather bold attempt at regulation had little impact on overall costs (Rimmer and Ross 1997), which increased by approximately 80 per cent between 1983 and 1993 (Central Statistical Office 1994), and substantially less than the amount claimed (Ryan and Yule 1993). The government's armoury was otherwise limited; it had no readily apparent means of influencing prescribing behaviour or holding GPs to account for the resources used in general practice. More fundamentally, the political agenda for general practice had not matured sufficiently: primary care had escaped the close attention of government, which had instead focused on the hospital sector. This was as true of the first half of the 1980s as it had been in previous decades.

This neglect ended, however, with the publication of a consultation paper *Primary Health Care: An Agenda for Discussion* (DHSS 1986), which listed among its aims a concern to improve standards, to achieve value for money and to create clearer priorities for FPSs. The subsequent White Paper *Promoting Better Health* (DHSS 1987) confirmed these objectives and defined a more assertive role for FPCs in the management of primary care, requiring a greater accountability of GPs. The two major policy instruments that would assist FPCs in this were the renegotiated GP contract and the NHS and Community Care Act 1990.

A description of the 1990 contract is provided in Chapter 3. For the purposes of this discussion, it is important to note that the explicitness of the contract, which set out in more precise terms than before what was required, was an important element in holding GPs to account (Petchey 1996). For example, the terms of service governing the availability of a GP were more clearly defined, requiring that full-time GPs made themselves available for five days in any working week and 'in such a manner as is likely to be convenient to his patients' (GMS 1992:49). In addition to specifying more precisely the service required of GPs, the contract linked some aspects of general medical services to performance. This transformed previous arrangements whereby GPs had been paid for immunisation and vaccination and cervical screening services on a fee-per-item basis, instead requiring GPs to achieve a target number of patients treated before payment was triggered. Upper and lower targets were also specified, additional rewards being reflected in payments for reaching the upper target. Health promotion clinics, an aspect of GP work previously unrewarded, henceforth attracted payment.

The lack of specificity in the contract and the absence of cash limits initially led to much additional activity of uncertain value (Paris *et al.* 1992), but more clearly defined criteria for health promotion payments were subsequently introduced (Chapter 3). The contract was not, however, entirely about patient service specifications. In a move that supported the RCGP's position on life-long education, it promoted regular postgraduate education by offering financial incentives to undertake training broadly equivalent to one week's course per year. This inducement will become a requirement if mandatory reaccreditation is introduced by either the profession or the state. This is probable given public and government disquiet over recent well-publicised failures of professional performance.

The 1990 contract was a watershed in the relations between GPs and the state. To begin with, it was imposed on an embittered medical workforce following a breakdown in negotiations between the representative bodies and the then Secretary of State for Health, Kenneth Clarke. The corporatism that had characterised historical dealings between state and profession had been abruptly terminated. As yet unable or unwilling to introduce competition into general practice, the government terminated the previous, rather *laissez-faire*, agreement with minimalist conditions of performance, which had been a barometer of the state's confidence in the professional model of accountability. It was replaced by a more prescriptive contract that not only sought to direct professional activity and encourage performance through financial incentives, but also, more assertively, expressed minimum standards of performance.

Although policy had to some extent been informed by professional debates, the broad direction in which the GPs' performance was being steered being consistent with the preferences of the academic leadership of the profession, the government defined the terms. Even though the measures introduced in the 1990 contract constituted only a restrained attempt to direct performance, they reflected a determination on the part of government to trespass on hallowed ground. The stratagems to manipulate clinical performance were modest. They were still broadly framed in terms of quantity rather than quality[3] and did not prescribe standards of care for certain conditions, but they intervened in the way in which GPs managed at-risk practice populations, and they established a precedent. The symbolic importance of this far outweighed any operational success.

The more robust 1990 contract did provide the newly constituted FHSAs with criteria by which the performance of GPs could be judged and improved. FHSAs themselves constituted an evolutionary progression from FPCs, which Huntingdon (1993) characterised as being managerially distanced from the DoH. From April 1991, FHSAs became accountable to regional health authorities for performance targets, which included improving standards of quality and cost-effectiveness in general practice. Although still one stage removed, the accountability of GPs was locked into the NHS structure. As Huntingdon makes clear, however, the leverage that FHSAs could apply was limited. As a last resort, FHSAs could discipline aberrant GPs who had failed to meet the conditions of service with reprimands and/or by withholding payments, and, in possible cases of professional misconduct, by referral to the GMC. Other than the disagreeable and professionally damaging consequences associated with these processes, the mechanisms available to FHSAs were financial. Apart from payments triggered by targets, the discretionary use of practice development monies constituted a useful, if limited, form of behaviour therapy.

If the broad mandate given to FHSAs was to improve standards of general practice, controlling the rate of increase in prescribing costs, and within this encouraging cost-effective prescribing habits, has been a particular concern. After 1991, FHSAs (subsumed within health authorities after 1996) indicated annual expenditure guidelines for practices (Indicative Prescribing Amounts [IPAs]), and GPs received quarterly reviews of their prescribing practices and associated costs. Some FHSAs mimicked the incentives found in the fundholding package and allowed non-fundholding practices that expended less than their IPA to invest the difference in practice infrastructure (Audit Commission 1994). Overprescribing practices may have been subject to sanctions in the form of withholding remuneration, but health authorities were more likely to value good relations with practices, preferring a more emollient approach. More commonly, health authorities deployed medical advisers. These were usually former GPs who encouraged change through education and persuasion, one element of which involved comparisons with the prescribing performance of other local practices. Thus, within the broadly managerialist model of accountability are to be found strategies that fit more appropriately within the professional model of accountability.

The Economic Model

It may well be that Conservative governments ultimately placed their faith in a consumerist model of accountability to secure an improvement in services rather than achieving this via audit and regulation by the profession or by direct management. The purchaser–provider division may have enhanced peer accountability, but of hospital clinicians to GPs rather than vice versa. In addition, the threat if not the reality of competition gave trust managers additional leverage over clinicians to improve output, even if not clinical outcome. Pressure to improve the quality of care was to be applied by informed providers who were GP fundholders or health authorities advised by public health doctors and GPs. Indirectly, therefore, GP fundholders were responsible, as purchasers, for securing improvements in secondary care, but there were no attempts to assess their performance in a routine way, far less to hold them to account formally.

There was, however, an isolated exception: *Working for Patients* (DoH 1990) had extended the remit of the Audit Commission to include the NHS as well as local government, and *What the Doctor Ordered* (Audit Commission 1996), despite its rather indulgent title, represented the Audit Commission's first major foray into the domain of general practice. It found that few fundholders reviewed clinical audit information or stipulated the approach that providers should take to ensuring effective treatment. Perhaps the latter inactivity was fortuitous since neither did most fundholders 'make full use of the increasing body of knowledge about clinical effectiveness' (1996:26). Nor was the performance of health authorities outstanding. Although their purchasing strategies were supposed to be informed by evidence-based medicine (NHSME 1991a, 1991b), in some health authorities other priorities, such as the waiting list initiative, vied for attention on purchasing agendas (Godber 1995, North 1998).

Despite this, the greater encouragement of fundholders, and to a lesser extent non-fundholders, to participate in strategic commissioning probably encouraged more evidence-based purchasing and, in the process, increased GPs' accountability for the delivery of national priorities. Overall, however, there was little evidence of health authorities' attempts to appraise systematically the success of fundholders as purchasers. This was a task left to the Audit Commission (1996) and to external researchers, for example Surender *et al.* (1995), who found that fundholders' referral rates to more expensive secondary care were not reduced compared with non-fundholding practices. Such research cannot, by its nature, be used to hold individual general practices to account, and where health authorities executed tentative evaluations of fundholder purchasing performance, they constituted a part of the repertoire of strategies within a managerial rather than an economic model of accountability.

Government policy was designed to appeal to fundholders as the rational/economic as opposed to professional 'man', but as far as the performance of GP fundholders was concerned, financial incentives in the form of fund savings, rather than competition and the feeble threat of exit by consumers (patients), were the inducements to change. Fundholders were accountable to FHSAs for the financial probity of funds, and practice accountability was increased, as health authorities demanded more information in order to monitor contracts. There were no clinical performance measures applied to fundholders beyond those incorporated into the new contract for all GPs. Such evidence as did exist focused on economic (cost) rather than clinical outcomes and was generated by research that anonymised the results. For example, Harris and Scrivenor (1996) observed that fundholders' prescribing was less costly than that of non-fundholders, but savings were greatest in the first year and declined thereafter. The poverty of the government's attempt rigorously to evaluate fundholding's performance may reflect the infancy of such projects in UK health care, although it is hardly credible that performance measures could not have been developed had government willed it so. A more probable explanation lies in a government reluctance to deter recruits to fundholding with the threat of external audit or, in the event of unsatisfactory outcomes, to provide fuel for critics of fundholding.

Had the Conservatives remained in office after the May 1997 election, accountability to health authorities for general medical services may well have been enhanced by competition between traditional general practices and commercial or community trust-run primary care services employing salaried GPs (DoH 1996b). Health authorities would thereby have become purchasers rather than contractors of services with local professional cartels. It is difficult to determine whether further recourse to the market, as a means of imposing greater control over doctors' clinical performance, would have been successful. The grip of government on clinical activity, particularly in relation to cost-effective care, has been tentative when compared with the USA's more closely regulated health care system and especially in relation to GPs, but this may be about to change.

Locking General Practice into a New NHS

The New NHS (DoH 1997) put an end to fundholding and in its place created PCGs or PCTs. Scotland and Wales have separate arrangements, which retain more control over commissioning for the respective Health Boards and health authorities (see Chapter 4). Proposals for Northern Ireland[4] are potentially the most radical of all but await a political settlement. It was always assumed that, in England, GPs would have a major role in the PCGs, but in the months following the publication of the White Paper, GP leadership lobbied hard for control of the PCGs' and a separation of the Hospital and Community Health Service's (HCHS) prescribing and practice infrastructure allocations.[5] PCGs and PCTs are accountable to health authorities for the execution of duties framed by targets for 'improving health, health services and value for money' (DoH 1997:Section 5.24). The involvement of all GPs, via their representatives, in PCG commissioning decisions, together with unified budgets, will significantly tighten GPs' accountability, not only as commissioners of services, but also as providers. In Scotland, the LHCCs (cooperatives of GPs) within SPCTs and the Welsh LHGs (broadly equivalent to stage 1 PCGs) may also be allocated budgets covering primary care services, although local circumstances will dictate the degree to which this occurs.

The most ambitious design for general practice, in England, reflects a complex, multilayered conceptualisation of accountability. It employs not only a managerial model of accountability – of PCG boards to health authorities, and GP members to the PCG board – but also requires professional accountability of member GPs to each other and, almost by default rather than design, limited political accountability. Since PCGs have to make decisions about service priorities, there is already a recognition that the local community will need to be consulted over decisions (Chisholm 1998), although recent research has suggested that GPs appear reluctant to become actively involved in PCG processes (North *et al.* 1999). A more obvious form of accountability is that to peers. In that GPs are responsible for the use of resources through prescribing and referral decisions, which, if overindulgent, may compromise resources for other services, practices or patients, there is likely to be an insistence from GPs that practice-level activity is closely monitored and maverick practices disciplined, possibly by limiting future allocations. Such disciplinary protocols would need to be negotiated with practices and established early in the life of PCGs before cases arise.

The interest in monitoring GP performance is likely to evolve into something more than an immediate concern with overshooting budgets. Variations in prescribing and referral habits will inevitably focus attention on individual or GP group professional practice. There is likely to be pressure to conform to guidelines endorsed by the PCG but configured nationally by the NICE and the National Service Frameworks. Scotland's LHCCs will no doubt have to respond to the equivalent, the proposed Health Technology Assessment Centre (Scottish Office 1997). The Commission for Health Improvement in England will not automatically review clinical governance within PCGs and PCTs, but the latter will be able to invite the Commission to examine problem services 'provided by their members as contractor professionals' (DoH 1998b:Section 4.25). The waters will be muddied as community trusts are already advertising for salaried GPs to operate in underserviced areas, and GP practices may in future be subcontracted by PCTs to undertake non-core general practice activities. It is unlikely, therefore, that PCG/PCTs can insist on specific standards of general practice without applying them internally.

The overall impression of *A First Class Service*, the DoH's (1998b) proposals for improving clinical and service quality in the NHS, was that a more pluralistic development of national standards for treatments and services would increasingly define clinical activity and service performance in primary care as well as the hospital sector. The profession read the runes and, in February 1999, moved to recapture the initiative. The GMC announced that doctors would have to submit to performance monitoring. General practices will now be required to produce a profile of each doctor, to include regular appraisal. The ultimate sanction for failing doctors is removal from the register. This move may have been successful in pre-empting government intervention in self-regulation but only at the 'cost' of pushing the profession to do more than it otherwise might have contemplated.

Conclusion

In 1992, three American academics, undoubtedly with the benefit of national hindsight, warned the readership of the *British Medical Journal* that 'no door bolts tightly enough to exclude the realities that have come to besiege modern medicine' (Berwick *et al.* 1992:235). Hospital clinicians and to a lesser extent GPs were presumably by then already aware of a changing political and organisational environment that had increasingly sought to monitor what doctors did and hold them accountable for their performance. The 1980s and 90s have seen a number of policy initiatives that have attempted to direct professional activity using peer pressure, rewards, regulation or the threat of sanctions to induce changes. These initiatives, which have not only used GPs to improve the performance of hospital clinicians, but also attempted to make GPs more accountable for services provided in general practice and ultimately the clinical practice of GPs themselves, are of critical importance. Collectively, they signify a loss of confidence in, although not a total rejection of, the professional model of accountability and recourse to external forms of regulation.

Recent proposals from the Blair government suggest a continuation of this approach, albeit one that relies less on the sanction of the market. A reliance on the exclusory professional model of accountability is eschewed in favour of a more open system that incorporates economic and patient perspectives in establishing benchmarks for acceptable performance and opens up clinical activity as well as service delivery to the gaze of the state. PCGs and, one level down, general practices will be accountable to health authorities for their performance in achieving stated goals; aberrant practice, to be similarly defined by externally generated criteria, will attract some form of sanction. The profession has tried to recapture the initiative by promoting self-regulatory practices, endeavours that are likely to continue for as long as there is a perceived challenge to professional autonomy. However, public and political confidence having been breached, the threat of state intervention is not likely to recede. Although as a consequence the profession may well strengthen internal regulation more than it might have been inclined to, this is unlikely to appease. If, for the present, '[medical] practitioners see their main channels of accountability to their peers' (Pratt 1995), they are unlikely to do so for long.

Notes

1. Following the postoperative deaths of 29 children, the GMC struck off a retired consultant cardiac surgeon and a retired former chief executive of the trust, and banned a second surgeon from carrying out paediatric heart surgery for three years. The same evening on a BBC television programme, Frank Dobson, the then Secretary of State for Health, was critical of the GMC's decision, stating that all three should have been removed from the register. The subsequent conviction of a Manchester GP for the murder of a number of elderly patients underlined concerns about the effectiveness of peer regulation.
2. A discouragement to divulge information about colleagues' poor performance was reinforced by a professional code that forbade doctors to disparage 'the professional skill, knowledge, qualifications or services of any other doctor' (GMC regulations, cited by Stacey 1992).
3. This claim is qualified by a consideration of such items as the specification of GP availability and the 'quality' outcomes associated with the achievement of population immunity by immunisation and vaccination, and the increased detection of cervical carcinoma.
4. Proposals in Northern Ireland, still to be introduced, are for five Health and Social Care Partnerships, each constituted from a number of Primary Care Cooperatives covering between 50,000 and 100,000 head of population. The Primary Care Cooperatives will be similar to PCGs but will hold budgets for social as well as health care, reflecting current organisational arrangements in Northern Ireland.
5. Items contained in a letter to Alan Milburn, Minister of Health, from Dr John Chisholm, Chairman of the General Medical Services Committee, which was circulated to BMA members in June 1998.

6

Practices and Patients

This chapter is the first of a pair that focus on matters concerning the location of general practices and their associated patients. The general theme for this first chapter is the relationship between general practice and deprivation. As primary first-stop providers of medical care, GPs directly experience the effects of the association between ill-health and the material living conditions of their patients. From the patient's perspective, general medical care should be available when needed. The evidence suggests, however, that what is available in and to deprived communities differs considerably from that in more affluent areas. These issues matter because the NHS has, from its inception, had a commitment to equality. Furthermore, contemporary New Labour health policy carries a commitment to the eradication of inequality, not least because of the role that more equitably available services may play in bringing about improvements in national health status.

There are two main sections to this chapter. In the first, consideration is given to the 'big picture'. The spotlight is placed on inequalities in the provision of general practice care at the national level. The extent of inequality in GP provision between regional divisions is considered, and policies designed to ensure equity in the distribution of GP services are outlined and evaluated. The second section looks at general practice and its patients on a more localised scale. It considers the relationship between inequality and deprivation, and reflects on mechanisms for rewarding GPs who serve deprived areas. As a prelude to these two more substantial sections, the chapter begins with a brief examination of some relevant general concepts and background matter.

Concepts and Background

Any discussion of deprivation and (in)equality begs questions about the nature of the issues under discussion. To clarify matters for this chapter, this section considers why inequality and deprivation are features that demand attention in any study of general practice. It also briefly outlines the key concepts that will be employed in the subsequent discussions.

At root, inequalities in the provision of general practice are manifestations of the impact of choice. People choose GPs, and GPs choose where they will practice. Both choices are heavily constrained and interrelated. An individual's choice of GP is constrained by the available supply of GPs, and a GP's choice of practice location is constrained by the availability of vacancies and patients. Taking patient choice first, it is evident that patients do not always register with their nearest GP, although most do. They may choose a GP near their work as opposed to their home. They may stay with a particular GP when they move house. Some individuals choose GPs on the basis of wanting a GP of a particular age, sex or ethnic group. These issues will be explored in more depth in the next chapter in the context of a discussion of the differences between general practice in rural and urban areas. More important in this present chapter are issues of GP choice regarding location. It is these GP choices which condition what is available to the public and where it is available.

Evidence about contemporary GP locational decision-making suggests the relevance of a number of factors. The UK situation with a national health service differs somewhat from that prevailing in other countries where one important factor may be the quality of the relationship between the GP and the local hospital and the associated spin-offs for effective and smooth referral from primary to secondary care. In such cases, proximity to a hospital is also an important factor. Of more relevance in the UK are personal factors (Wilkin *et al.* 1987). GPs tend to settle in areas close to the medical school at which they trained. They prefer practices in pleasant residential environments as they usually like to live relatively close to the practice. Many cite family reasons, including a family practice tie or the presence of elderly relatives in an area. Some doctors may move to be near their partner's job. Although there are exceptions, it is also the case that GPs tend to hope to practise in areas that will, on average, be less likely to generate high levels of demand and particularly unpredictable demand. Alongside these personal factors lie those associated with the supply of GPs and the supply of land and funding for building surgeries. Few GPs still in active practice would have had to take whatever opening was available when they graduated. This was, however, certainly an issue for GPs in the early years of the NHS. Land supply factors that used to ensure that GP practices were to be found in areas where there was a supply of larger houses for conversion now ensure that new premises are in locations where new-build is possible.

The outcome of these GP locational decision-making processes is that there is a clear geography to the provision of general practice. The consequent question is: are these GPs in the right places? Distributional justice as a research area has a long pedigree (Powell 1990, 1995). Davies' (1968) work provides a useful point of departure for the perspectives in this chapter. Territorial justice should be a situation in which provision is located where it is needed. It allows that some areas may have quantitatively more than others in so far as they may *need* more than others. This distinction between simple provision and provision in relation to need is usually summarised as a distinction between equality and equity. Where equity does not prevail, the situation is known as inverse care (Tudor Hart 1971). Although it might be argued that inverse care in general practice is an inevitable consequence of the free choice of GPs, the empirical identification of inverse care is seldom simple. As Powell (1990) notes, past research on the topic has been the subject of varying methods, and testing has not been standardised or even very well carried out.

The National Picture

As might be surmised from Chapter 2, the NHS inherited what Wilkin *et al.* (1987:2) rightly termed 'a patchwork of service provision, much of it distinguishable only by degrees of awfulness'. For the reasons suggested in the previous section, the provision of general practice tended to be lower in more working-class areas. The early NHS was thus characterised by what Powell (1997:35) terms the 'geography of affluence':

> doctors were more strongly associated with areas of high rateable value and low infant mortality... the county boroughs, the resorts and spas – the so-called watering holes – or the 'bath chair towns' had the most doctors while the poorer areas had least.

This distributional geography largely mirrored what had been the situation in the late 1930s (PEP 1944). Although Powell (1992) sees the Political and Economic Planning Report as a flawed offering, it is clear that, while the provision of GPs varied sevenfold across the country as a whole, there was substantially less variation between some areas, most notably between shire and county boroughs, and substantially more within other areas, particularly London.

Elements of this distributional geography of general practice have persisted through over 50 years of an NHS committed to equality of access. Some 30 years after the birth of the NHS, Knox (1979) used location quotients for the old (pre-1995) regional health authorities (Health Boards in Scotland) to show that the South West, South East and East Anglia, and most of Scotland apart from the urban west and Fife, had more GPs than they should have done on the basis of their population alone.

Figure 6.1 shows the contemporary picture. It is evident that, on the simple basis of the number of GPs per 100,000 people, there is now consider-

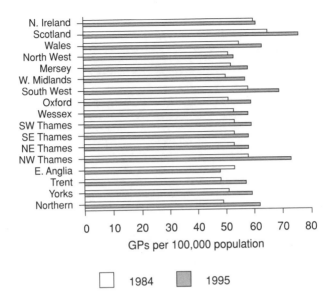

Figure 6.1   GP provision by region; 1984 and 1995, per 100,000 people

able equality between the regions of England, Wales and Northern Ireland. There do, however, remain a number of exceptions to this generalisation. There are significantly more GPs per 100,000 people in Scotland, in the South West and in the North West Thames area. There are also significantly fewer in East Anglia. It is worth noting, however, that this distributional geography is volatile. Not only does it run counter to that found by Knox some 25 years ago, but it is also different from that prevailing 10 years ago. As Figure 6.1 shows, the relative equality of the mid-1990s masks the greater degree of equality that existed in the early 1980s. The higher levels of provision evident in 1995 were still higher but less markedly so in 1984. East Anglia appears to be the only region that has actually seen a reducing level of per capita provision.

Designated Areas Policy

Figure 6.2 examines the issue of regional equality in GP provision in a slightly different way. The number of GPs as a fraction of the population of an area does not take account of the fact that a proportion of the population do not

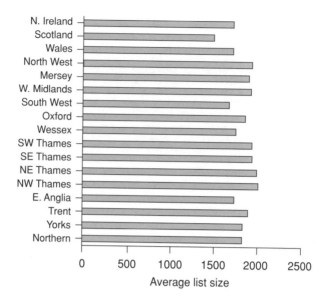

Figure 6.2   GP average list size, 1995, by region

register with a GP. List size, on the other hand, does make the registration issue explicit and thus provides a basic indication of the relative disparity in GP workload across the UK. Again, a considerable degree of equality is evident, and, as expected, list sizes appear lowest in Scotland. They are not, however, highest in East Anglia; in general, the higher values are in the more urbanised areas of the South East (the Thames regions) and the Mersey–North West. Over the past 10 years, there has been a small but clear reduction in GP list size across all regions.

List size inequalities have formed the basis of the main policy instrument designed to address inequalities in GP provision. The Medical Practice Committees (MPCs) set up at the start of the NHS have regulated provision by reference to the average list size within defined medical practice areas (MPAs), of which there are around 1,450 in England and Wales. The idea of the policy was to provide financial incentives to attract personnel to under-doctored areas (where list sizes were high) and set up sanctions to limit recruitment or impose quotas elsewhere, particularly where list sizes were unusually low. The policy was initially based on MPAs being subdivisions of FHSAs. Later, they became subdivisions of health authorities, and, as of 1998, the plan was that they would be realigned to ensure co-terminosity with PCGs in recognition of the fact that the envisaged optimum size of a PCG

Table 6.1 Medical practice area classification

Area type	Restricted	Intermediate	Open	Designated
Average list size	0–1,700	1,700–2,100	2,100–2,500	2,500+

(100,000 residents) had long been recognised by the MPC as also being the optimum size for an MPA.

MPA policy has worked by classifying MPAs into groupings based on average list size. There were originally three types of area: designated, intermediate and restricted. In designated areas, list sizes were high and new GPs were welcomed. The replacement of a retiring GP was usually a matter of course in an intermediate area. Restricted areas had low list sizes, and new GPs were normally not allowed either to form a new practice or to replace a retiring GP. Over time, the policy saw a number of changes. From 1962 onwards, the 'intermediate grade' was separated into two, the automatic replacement of a retiring GP being allowed in a new grade of 'open' area. In 1966, alongside the package of measures instituted as part of the 1965/66 GP contract, financial inducements were put in place to encourage GPs to (re)locate to designated areas. The designated area allowance was on a sliding scale designed to reflect the degree of under-doctoring within an MPA. It was payable as a salary supplement. Both in 1975 and in 1981, the criteria used to apply the now fourfold classification of MPAs were changed. The classification that now applies is set out in Table 6.1.

Three points need to be made about Table 6.1 that are not immediately evident. First, there are currently no designated areas (MPC 1998). The last, in County Durham, was eliminated in February 1986, at which time 75 per cent of England and Wales was classified as restricted or intermediate (Jones and Moon 1987). Second, there have been no areas officially classed as open since September 1997. The number of open areas had fallen to around 40 by the mid-1980s, at which time the MPC undertook a review jointly with the health authorities to identify means of reducing average lists and recruiting more GPs to open areas. This review assisted the further reduction of the number of open areas. Known health authority plans for increasing GP numbers have resulted in the creation of a subcategory of 'artificially intermediate' in 26 MPAs where developments should ensure that areas that would otherwise be open will soon become intermediate. These areas are being kept under review. The third point to note concerning Table 6.1 is that designated and open areas have been traditionally thought of as having an insufficient provision of GPs, that is, they are 'under-doctored'. Restricted areas are, in contrast, regarded as more than adequately doctored. The MPC does not subscribe to the view that the disappearance of designated and open areas means there is no longer anywhere in England and Wales where there is an insufficiency of GPs. It claims that the present situation is indicative of equality rather than adequacy (MPC 1998).

Butler *et al.* (1973) provide the classic study of MPA policy in action. They suggest that the MPA policy was initially very effective but that this effectiveness should be seen in the context of a good supply of new GPs and very few vacancies, a situation that led many newly qualified doctors in the late 1940s and 50s to take whatever vacancy arose or set up new practices in areas that were under-doctored and where patient lists could be built up more easily. This position came to an end with the crisis of general practice in the late 1950s and early 1960s, when newly qualified doctors drifted away from general practice towards hospital medicine and an undersupply of potential GPs resulted. The Office for Health Economics (1966) reported that, in the mid-1960s, the number of designated areas had doubled to approximately 35 per cent of all MPAs. The situation worsened in the late 1960s and continued through the 1970s as the supply of GPs failed to keep up with population growth (Knox 1978). Butler *et al.* (1973) noted a slight drop in the number of designated areas in the years immediately preceding their study, although they indicated that the number of such areas still accounted for some 20 per cent of MPAs as they went to publication. Furthermore, they found substantial geographical variations in the distribution of designated areas. Fully two-thirds of the old West Midlands Regional Health Authority was designated, while the corresponding figure was less than 8 per cent in the South West. Butler and his colleagues ultimately ended up questioning the extent to which MPA policy had, by 1973, brought about a real reduction in inequality of provision. Although quantitative disparities had changed for the better, the broad pattern of underprovision had not significantly changed in 30 years.

Figure 6.3 summarises what has happened to designated, open and restricted areas since the Butler research. The effect of the 1981 revision of the classification criteria is clear, as is the decline in the number of GPs practising in designated and open areas. There is also an evident rise in the number of restricted areas. The closure of restricted areas to new GPs has long been welcomed by existing GPs in such areas as it protects them from further competition. The major growth area, the rise in the number of GPs practising in intermediate areas, is not shown as the number involved is an order of magnitude larger. It is this absent line on the graph which is perhaps the most significant in terms of (in)equality as it signifies the considerable extent to which there is now a remarkably even distribution of GPs across England and Wales.

It is difficult to ascribe a precise cause-and-effect linkage that would give sole or even the majority of the credit for the claimed current equality of provision of GPs to MPA policy; GP supply factors have undoubtedly played

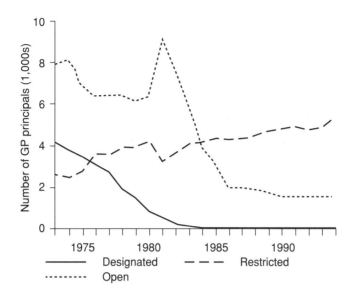

Figure 6.3 Medical practice areas, 1973–94

at least as important a role. Furthermore, as noted above, the MPAs have changed in terms of their classification over the years in which the policy has been operational. Additionally, the number of MPAs has also changed, as have their boundaries. There has been a policy of amalgamating smaller MPAs into larger units, the details of which practices and which communities are covered by which MPA often having been a well-kept secret.

While these factors cast some statistical fog over the apparent success of MPA policy, rather more significance can, however, be attached to a more fundamental limitation. As the previous section indicated, there is a difference between equality and equity. MPA policy has historically been based only on average list size; it has been concerned with equality but not with equity. There has been no attempt to assess the extent to which a variation in list size might be an acceptable reflection of underlying differences in the need for health care. Nor does the patient list measure give any indication of the quality of what is being provided. Recent developments are seeking to address this issue, most notably through the construction of adjustment factors to lists to take account of deprivation and other factors that may, to some extent, justify smaller lists.

At best, therefore, MPA policy is a crude instrument which, as Powell (1990) has remarked, makes the crucial assumption that all patients have equal needs and that all GPs are of equal quality and undertake equal workloads. In fact, the general decline of list size over time has been such that the policy has shifted from being one in which GPs were encouraged to practise in under-doctored areas, however imperfectly identified, to one of negative direction, preventing people setting up rather than encouraging them.

Workloads and Deprivation

This section focuses down from the big picture of national variations in GP distribution and the policies put in place to counter such inequalities. The emphasis is now on more local relationships between general practice and the issue of deprivation. In particular, attention turns to an examination of the extent to which some GPs serve a disproportionate number of deprived patients. Embodied in this concern is the need to reflect upon the frequent conflation of deprivation with workload.

The underlying rationale for studying the extent to which GPs serve deprived patients stems from the massively influential conclusions of the Black Report on health inequalities (DHSS 1980, Townsend and Davidson 1988). The Black Report suggested that there was a strong and causal association between material deprivation, and ill-health and mortality. It also identified a clear interaction between social and geographical factors as an underpinning to patterns of morbidity and mortality. The effect of these relationships and associations was that poorer people living in poorer housing conditions and less favourable socio-economic circumstances were more likely to be suffering from ill-health and dying younger. They were also more likely, as a consequence, to consult their GP more frequently, albeit often less effectively. By extension, GPs serving deprived patients were more likely to have higher workloads and face greater clinical need. In short, therefore, in the context of general practice, extra workload and the presence of deprivation are synonymous. Deprivation is not only important in its own right, but is also symptomatic of the difficulties of delivering care and thus indicative of probable extra costs of provision.

To plan effectively for this increased activity would require data on the social characteristics of patients, which are not generally available. Where they have been collected, for example by a general practice, they are seldom in a standardised form and are governed by restrictive confidentiality constraints. In the absence of individual data on patients, an alterative strategy is required. This takes the form of ecological surrogacy: the characteristics of a geographical area are assumed to apply to all the people living in that area. On the one hand, this strategy solves the problem: data from the decennial population census are available in some considerable detail for small areas and, while these data do not cover morbidity other than in the form of counts of people suffering limiting long-term illness, they provide a great deal of information on socio-economic factors that have been regularly and conclusively shown to be related to ill-health. On the other hand, as will be discussed later, the strategy runs the risk of the aggregative fallacy by assuming that the characteristics of an area are shared by all its inhabitants. This is manifestly not always the case: within any one deprived area there are likely to be a number of individuals who are not themselves deprived.

Despite this difficulty, the population census has been widely used as the basis for studies of deprivation and general practice. Measuring deprivation using the census has a long and varied pedigree. It is possible to use single census variables, such as a count of the population seeking work (unemployed) or, to adjust for varying population denominators, a percentage of such indicators. More often, however, multivariable indices are used. These form the basis of what Curtis and Taket (1997:148) have described as a 'mushrooming of research on small area indicators'. They typically employ a standard score (Z-score) transformation to adjust a number of indicators to a common scale. The various transformed indicators are then summed to provide a single composite indicator.

It was precisely this process which was followed in the calibration of perhaps the best-known multivariable composite index of deprivation in the general practice arena: the 'Jarman index', also known as the 'underprivileged area' (UPA) index and the Jarman 8 or UPA 8 after the number of variables involved. Building on work originally commissioned by the Acheson Review of Primary Health Care in Inner London (LHPC 1981; see Chapter 7), this index focused on GP workload. The first stage of the research was to ask a 1 in 10 national sample of GPs to list the population subgroups that they felt contributed most to GP workload (Jarman 1983). They were given a list of 13 social factors and eight 'service factors' to prompt their responses (Table 6.2). These prompts were culled from an analysis of some 370 replies to a call for comments on issues affecting GP workload issued in the London area as part of the Acheson Review. The listing was conducted on the basis of GPs' own experiential conclusions but bore out much of what is known of the key characteristics of people who use general practice the most. As far as the social factors are concerned, there is a considerable overlap with those groups identified in more extensive empirical studies as being the most frequent users of general practice (Morell *et al.* 1971, McCormick *et al.* 1995, Neal *et al.* 1998; see also Chapter 1). A total of 2,614 questionnaires were sent as part of the national study, and 1,802 replies were usable for analytical purposes.

In the ensuing analysis, it was decided to concentrate on social factors alone, the last three social factors being discarded. Unmarried couples with families probed the same construct as lone parenthood, while crime and vandalism and difficulties visiting defied easy measurement in so far as they were not readily available as census indicators. This left a set of 10 indicators,

Table 6.2   Jarman index: initial prompts

Social factors	Service factors
Older people (aged 65+)	Long outpatient waiting times
Children aged under 5	Low expenditure on community services relative to hospital services
Unemployment	
Poor housing	Low expenditure on social services
People born outside the UK	Low number of nurses attached to general practices
Single-parent households	
Elderly living alone	Many elderly GPs
Overcrowding	Many single-handed GPs
Lower social class	High GP list size
High household mobility	Low GP list size
Unmarried couples with families	
Crime and vandalism	
Difficulty visiting	

N.B. The terminology has been slightly adjusted to reflect current equivalencies.

which was subsequently rationalised to eight (Jarman 1984). Poor housing, measured as the number of households lacking access to basic amenities such as an indoor toilet, was dropped as it was no longer sufficiently common to enable the identification of a significant fraction of the households in the country, nor was it a particularly useful indicator as many houses were thought to be in a poor state of repair despite possessing basic amenities. The over-65 population was also discarded as it duplicated the elderly living alone indicator without having the same discriminatory power. Each of the final selection of indicators was assigned a weight reflecting the relative importance ascribed by the national GP group. Table 6.3 provides details of the final indicators and their weighting.

The dropping of the service indicators reflected a number of factors. In the first place, they were open to manipulation. Unlike the social variables, it would have been possible for a health authority, or, at the time, an FPC, to allocate more resources or shift its pattern of expenditure and thus change its score on a service indicator. In essence, the service indicators identified a different component of workload, and the decision was taken to focus on those aspects of workload which were outside the control of the NHS. A second shortcoming of service indicators was that, even had they been chosen, the available data for their measurement would not allow a local-scale study, largely because they would not have been available from the

Table 6.3   The Jarman 8 (UPA 8) index

Indicator (all % of residents in private households)	Weight
Pensioners living alone	6.62
Children aged under five	4.64
Single-parent households	3.01
People in unskilled occupations	3.74
Unemployed people	3.34
People in overcrowded households	2.88
People moving house in the year before the census	2.68
People born in the New Commonwealth or Pakistan	2.50

population census. Indeed, for the purposes of the study of GP workload, they would have been singularly useless as most would only have been available for areas far larger than those served by an individual general practice. Third, many of the suggested service indictors were strongly interrelated, not only internally within the service indicator group, but also with the social indicators. Despite these cogent reasons for their omission, a note of caution must, however, be sounded. By deciding against service indicators, the Jarman index explicitly ignored the fact that a substantial element of GP workload is generated not by patients but by the NHS through bureaucratic demands, or by GPs themselves through recommending return consultations or giving unclear messages to patients (Armstrong *et al.* 1990).

The Jarman index has now effectively gone through three phases. The initial work was undertaken using the 1971 population census. Index figures were calculated for each of the London boroughs (Jarman 1983). The results were suggested to be a good match to expectations concerning the distribution of GP workload. The exercise was then extended to the rest of England and Wales down to a local government ward level using 1981 data. Initial testing took place in the Kensington, Chelsea and Westminster, Bedfordshire, Mid Glamorgan and Liverpool FPC areas (Jarman 1984). A parallel test was also run to derive a similar index for community nursing workloads (Jarman 1989). When the 1991 data became available, the index was again recalculated. The actual process of calculating the indicator involved five steps: conversion to percentages, a transformation to approximate statistical normality, standardisation using Z-scores, weighting and the final summation. Positive scores on the final index were indicative of an above-average workload, with a higher score equating to a higher workload. District health authority-level UPA scores using the 1981 data ranged from –32.79 to +54.89 (Tower Hamlets). Other district health authorities receiving low scores were

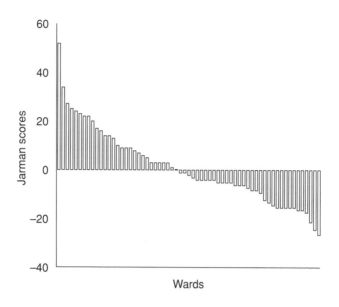

Figure 6.4   1991 Jarman scores – a case study district health authority

Central Manchester, City of London and Hackney, West Birmingham, Paddington and North Kensington, Camberwell, West Lambeth, Islington, Bradford and Newham (Jarman 1989). The preponderance of London health authorities in this list raised the question of a possible London bias in the index, to which we will return later.

Figure 6.4 shows the 1991-based ward-level UPA profile for one district health authority in southern England. The highest positive value is from an inner city area characterised by both a high percentage of elderly people living alone and a very high percentage of one-parent families. Its UPA score is among the highest in the country. Interestingly, however, and this is another point that will be returned to later, it has lower percentages of young children and overcrowding than the third-highest scoring ward, a large public sector overspill estate. Of the 10 highest scoring wards, only one could not be generally categorised as either inner city or overspill estate. In contrast, the wards with negative scores are private sector suburbs and rural areas.

Figure 6.5 shows the distribution of scores for the former FHSAs of England and Wales categorised by whether they are from shire counties, metropolitan counties, the Greater London area or Wales. Given that the national average Jarman score is, by definition, zero, there are some evident

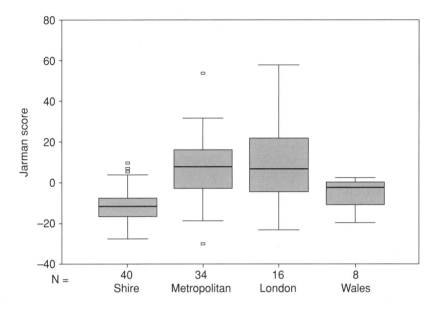

Figure 6.5   1991 Jarman scores – Family Health Services Authority level

variations by type of area. The highest scores are in metropolitan counties and in Greater London; both these types of area have, on average, a level of GP workload that is above the national mean.

There are a number of problems with the Jarman index, which can all be traced to three basic factors. First, the relationship between health and deprivation is geographically variable (Fox *et al.* 1984, Blaxter 1990, Eames *et al.* 1992) as well as varying over time (Bryce *et al.* 1994). It follows that the implications of deprivation for GP workload also vary over time and are not the same in all places. The Jarman index assumes that the same factors influence workload in all areas of the country and that their relative weighting has remained constant over time. While it is undeniable that a validation exercise was conducted, the concentration of high index values in London has led to allegations of a London focus, an urban emphasis and a persistent bias against northern areas (Leavey and Wood 1985, Senior 1991). It is equally undeniable that the index has been updated as new census data have become available. It is not, however, clear that the original weighting still remains valid. Nor is it clear that a common set of national weights is appropriate; the remarkable coincidence of weighting between urban and rural GPs noted in Jarman (1983) may not have been sustained.

A second set of drawbacks to the Jarman index concern its reliance on the census. The variables comprising the index clearly constrain the final form of the index, and this constraint is heightened by limiting the index to variables routinely available from the census. Different variables (as well as different or differential weighting) might generate very different results. The relatively high weighting given to elderly people living alone may, for example, be more appropriate in some areas than others. As will be seen below, the continued debate over the relative worth of the Jarman compared with other indices is further evidence of this problem. The census base also means that the index can be updated only on a 10-yearly basis. Nor is it clear that the index is sufficiently robust to accommodate the known deficiencies of the 1991 census. Majeed *et al.* (1996) note how that census suffered from limitations, with important implications for workload measurement, including the underenumeration and undercounting of homeless people and refugees.

Finally, the decision to limit the index to census variables yet employ a multivariable formulation also means that the final index actually mixes a number of quite distinct concepts. As Senior (1991) notes, some variables capture 'risk' (older people living alone) whereas others relate more to the volume of routine workload (children aged under five). Carr-Hill and Sheldon (1991) provide a reminder that, in focusing on census indicators, the index also fails to take account of the extent to which alternative services, such as social work, district nursing and health visiting can alleviate workload. They also recognise that there is a converse to the workload focus: practices also serve distributions of patients who do *not* generate workload.

Senior (1991) provides the most comprehensive critique of the statistical problems that arise from the Jarman index. This is the third problem area. Central to Senior's analysis is the degree of success enjoyed by the transformation and standardisation processes employed in the index construction. These should result in each of the component indicators having a distributional histogram that is statistically 'normal', that is, a bell-shaped curve. Examination of the components post-transformation reveals that this is not entirely achieved for any indicator. It is especially not achieved for the minority ethnic group indicator, where, even after transformation, there is a substantial skew towards wards with low values. This has the effect of inflating the Jarman score by imposing an additional unknown weight that brings a higher score to GPs with a higher proportion of patients born in the New Commonwealth or Pakistan. Senior also draws attention to the difficulties of using wards as the spatial basis of the index. Census enumeration districts would provide a finer grain of analysis more in keeping with the relatively fine distribution of deprivation within the population. Shifting to an enumeration district scale of analysis would, however, expose index calculation to further problems as, on the enumeration district scale, census data are subject to random minor adjustments to protect respondent confidentiality. A later analysis (Senior 1995) noted a further statistical problem: that of denominator variability. Wards vary very substantially in their population size. By weighting for denominator size, it is possible to take some account of the greater social heterogeneity present in larger wards.

The Jarman index has been widely tested for its relationship to other factors. Hutchinson *et al.* (1989), Curtis (1990), Cotgrove *et al.* (1992) and Jessop (1992) have all provided local attempts at validating its effectiveness as a measure of workload. Its utility in relation to other social indicators has been tested by Carr-Hill *et al.* (1996). These authors found that, when the characteristics of individual patients are known and controlled for, the role of the Jarman index as a useful measure of ward-level deprivation is considerably reduced. There are also suggestions that it correlates relatively well with limiting long-term illness and the rate of permanent sickness-based absence from work. Associations with measures of morbidity and mortality are also generally good. Charlton and Lakhani (1985) note a good correlation with the number of deaths from hypertension and stroke, and with deaths from, as well as diagnoses of, cervical cancer and tuberculosis.

Perhaps most interesting, however, in view of the decision to discard service factors from the index construction, is the relationship of the Jarman index to service measures. Jarman (1989) was able to link index scores with wards where there were higher GP–patient ratios. Buckingham and Freeman (1997) suggested that deprivation, as measured by the Jarman score, seemed to influence the use of district nursing, health visiting, chiropody, community maternity services, community mental illness provision, and professions allied to medicine. Hippisley-Cox *et al.* (1997) made adjustments for partnership size, fundholding status and the size of the elderly practice population and found a significant independent association between deprivation, as measured by the Jarman score, and high total and medical referral rates. The Jarman score alone explained 29 and 35 per cent of the variation in total and medical referral rates respectively. This association was most probably caused by a link with morbidity and deprivation, although Hippisley-Cox *et al.* recognised that it could also reflect differences in patients' perceptions of their need for follow-up care, differential behaviour on the part of GPs or the availability of secondary care services.

As has been suggested above, the Jarman index is not without its rivals. Three competing indices are frequently cited: the Townsend, Carstairs and Department of Environment indices. These competitors employ fewer variables and use different weights (or, in the case of the Townsend index, no weights). All are similarly based on census variables but all are arguably better measures of deprivation than that of Jarman, in which deprivation is defined in a strict sense and seen as being separate from workload. Dolan *et al.* (1995) compared intercensus change for the Jarman, Townsend and Carstairs scores calculated from the 1981 and 1991 census data. The national values of equivalent variables derived from the censuses were calculated and normalised on the same baseline of 1981 summary statistics. For England and Wales, the Jarman score increased by 5.62 units, but the Townsend and Carstairs scores fell by 2.39 and 1.13 units respectively. The implications of this finding are that Townsend and Carstairs are rather more successful at picking up general reductions in material deprivation while Jarman is less effective. This difference is in part accounted for by the fact that the Jarman index contains measures of family structure while the other indices do not, and levels of lone parenthood increased markedly during the 1980s. Carlisle and Johnstone (1998), in a study of 29,142 patients in North Nottinghamshire, confirmed that both the Townsend score and the Jarman score were associated with surgery consultation rates at ward level. The Townsend score, however had a stronger association than the Jarman score ($r^2 = 0.59$ as against $r^2 = 0.39$) because all four of its component variables were individually associated with increased consultations, compared with four out of the eight Jarman components.

Balarajan *et al.* (1992) provide a further twist to the process. Their index weighted differentially for different demographic groups and used seven census indicators. The weighting was based on GP consultations reported in the General Household Surveys of 1983–87. Odds ratios for GP consultations were obtained for the selected variables among children (0–15 years), men (aged 16–64), women (aged 16–64) and elderly people (65 years and over). These were then used to derive weighted deprivation indices specific to electoral wards for use in general practice. Council tenure significantly increased the likelihood of consultation significantly in all four groups. Odds ratios were raised in children, men and women with no access to a car. Birth in the New Commonwealth or Pakistan yielded a high odds ratio in men, women and elderly people but not in children. Marginally increased consultation rates were evident in the manual socio-economic groups in women, elderly people, and children with a single-parent mother. The deprivation indices for general practice derived using these odds ratios varied substantially among electoral wards, that of the electoral ward of Hulme, Greater Manchester, being 24 per cent higher than that of the average ward in England, and that of the Cheam South ward of Sutton, London, 11 per cent lower than average. A similar 'objective' weighting was proposed by Scott-Samuel (1984). Lloyd *et al.* (1995) proposed a further index at both FHSA and practice level based on the percentage of prescribed items exempt from the prescription charge under the low-income scheme. The ranking FHSAs on the new index correlated highly with rankings on other indices.

Deprivation Payments

Carr-Hill and Sheldon (1991) bemoan the lack of validation and the uncertainty over exactly what the Jarman index measures and means. The context of their paper is the remarkable metamorphosis from a measure of workload to an all-purpose pan-NHS indicator of deprivation that the Jarman index underwent at the start of the 1990s. Its big moment was heralded in the 1987 primary care White Paper (DHSS 1987). Paragraph 3.38 stated that 'The government will introduce a new allowance especially related to working in areas of deprivation'. It was then adopted as the basis for calibrating deprivation payments to GPs as part of the implementation of the 1990 GP contract.

The use of the Jarman index, an area-based measure, reflects the absence of socio-economic information on each patient and the consequent need to make the ecological assumption that people in deprived areas are deprived people and thus likely to generate more workload for GPs. Each patient on a GP's list is allocated to a local government ward by means of a postcode–ward linkage file. Payments are made in proportion to the number of patients that a GP has in a deprived ward. The definition of a 'deprived' ward is, however, contentious. As the 1990 contract noted, 'Within the group of wards that are categorised as deprived, some are significantly more deprived than others' (GB Departments of Health 1989). It was suggested that wards should be ranked, those with greater deprivation receiving a greater supplement. A sliding scale was promised. In practice, this 'tapering payment' approach was not adopted and, rather than deprivation being seen as a continuum from nil to high, it is seen in terms of a stepped series of thresholds. Deprived wards were classed as those with a Jarman score of over 50 (high), 40–50 (medium) or 30–40 (low). Latterly, an additional category of wards with scores in the range of 20–30 was added. Residents of the four classes of 'deprived' ward attract deprivation payments commensurate with the banding scheme. Using the 1981 version of the Jarman score (with the threefold banding), some 454 wards in England attracted some level of deprivation payment.

The 1991 version of the Jarman index sees about half of all GPs having patients who attract deprivation payments on their practice lists. In 1994, the highest proportion of GPs with patients in deprived areas was in Scotland (Figure 6.6). Overall, 10 per cent of the population live in wards that attract deprivation payments.

There are some significant differences between the regional distribution of GPs attracting deprivation payments and the distribution of the population in wards that attract deprivation payments, in large part reflecting geographical variations in the extent to which GPs are located close to deprived areas. Thus in Scotland, relatively few people live in wards that attract deprivation payments but the urban concentration of those wards and of GPs ensures that

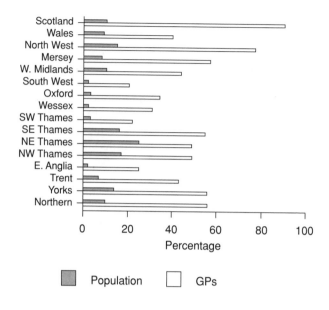

Figure 6.6   GPs with deprivation payments – population
attracting deprivation payments, 1994

a very high percentage of GPs have patients who attract some deprivation
payment. It is equally evident that regions such as the South West, Wessex,
Oxford and East Anglia have relatively few wards that attract deprivation
payments, nor do many GPs receive such payments.

Local-level analyses can substantiate these points. In the south of England
health authority case study used earlier, there are nine wards that attract
deprivation payments (having a Jarman score of over 20). In the most
deprived ward (with a Jarman score of 53.03), 37 GP practices serve the registered patient population. Six of these practices have over 1,000 patients and
account for half the ward's registered population. The remaining practices
share out the other half of the population, and some have only a few patients.
All 37, however, benefit to a greater or lesser extent from the high-level deprivation payments. Among the factors underpinning the relatively high
number of practices serving this deprived inner city area are the prevalence of
smaller size practices in inner city areas, the density and the mobility of the
population. Even those practices with substantial registered populations
within the deprived area also have patients in other wards. The practice with
most patients in the ward has nearly three times as many patients in other
wards. Neighbouring wards also attract deprivation payments, albeit at a

lower level, but there will also be patients who attract no deprivation payment. The relatively dispersed nature of GP practice populations means therefore that, in overall terms, many practices that attract deprivation payments also have a substantial patient population who are to be found in relatively less deprived areas. An indication of the effect of this phenomenon can be gauged by constructing practice-level Jarman scores.

Figure 6.7 shows such scores for the practices in the case study health authority. A comparison with Figure 6.4 above confirms the extent to which the scattered nature of practice patient lists leads to a less stark picture of deprivation. The differing length of the lines indicates that there are more practices than wards. The ward distribution of scores has a greater range and more perturbations. The practice scores bunch around the zero mark, and the gradient from most to least deprived is more shallow.

The crude stepped threshold approach to eligibility for deprivation payments inevitably excludes some practices and also makes the assumption that the resource consequences of deprivation impact at thresholds rather than in any other way (Senior 1991). This means that people in areas with scores just below the threshold bring no financial reward. This is patently unjust as well as being an unrealistic way to take account of the impact of deprivation on GP workload. Other problems with the present system of deprivation payments include its potential to act as a basis for exclusion and

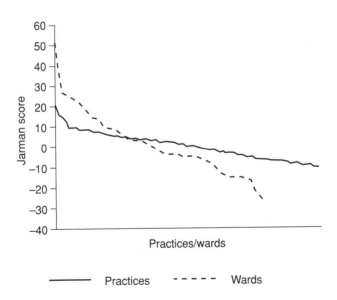

Figure 6.7   Ward and practice Jarman scores compared

its adequacy as a payment for extra workload. Baggott (1994:217) cites the case of two local authority housing estates in Carlisle that had a high positive Jarman score and had been deemed to be outside the area of one particular general practice. Baggott notes, however, that there was little evidence that such exclusion was widespread and further suggests that, for many practices, deprivation payments function as a form of compensation for low target payments for immunisation uptake. Worrall *et al.* (1997) assessed the adequacy of 'deprivation' payments in relation to actual costings for patients living in qualifying areas. Morbidity, workload and the costs of drug treatment were found to increase with decreasing socio-economic status. They suggested that deprivation payments met only half the extra workload cost for patients from qualifying wards and intimated that the payment system represented an inadequate incentive to encourage GPs to provide services in deprived areas.

Moore (1995) adds a more geographical point. He revisits the criticism that the Jarman index assumes that factors underlying deprivation (or workload) remain the same in all areas of the country. In reality, he notes, the precise manner in which the index was applied varied between the constituent parts of the UK. Only England uses the actual published version of the index. The application of the original index to Wales had resulted in only 10 wards being categorised as deprived, an outcome patently at odds with both the social and health conditions prevailing in the South Wales valleys and the former North East Wales coalfield. Housing variables were enhanced in Wales and a factor reflecting variations in standardised mortality ratios was introduced. In Scotland, postcode sectors were originally used but were later abandoned for enumeration districts, and the 'unskilled' variable was excluded. The 'ethnic' variable was dropped in Northern Ireland in recognition of the low level of minority ethnic group membership; lower cut-off points for deprivation payments were also instituted – had the original cut-off points been used, only 12 wards would have qualified for payments, again a situation at odds with the known health needs of Northern Ireland.

For Majeed *et al.* (1996), the validity of the current system of deprivation payments would be improved if data limitations were borne in mind when allocating payments to practices and if enumeration districts rather than electoral wards were used as the basis of payments. O'Reilly and Steele (1998) explore this issue as well as the question of a tapered relationship between funding and deprivation. They model three alternatives to the present system using Northern Ireland as an analytical base. Each of the three alternatives would redirect funds away from areas within the current payment bands towards those which previously failed to attract any deprivation payments. The loss would be greatest for those areas within the present 'low' payment band and least for those in the 'high' payment band. More equitable alternatives for allocating GP deprivation payments would thus lead to a significant movement of funds between areas. Hutchinson *et al.* (1989) and Senior (1991) reached a similar conclusion and also indicated that abandoning Jarman for Townsend would benefit Merseyside, Humberside and the North East at the expense of South and East London.

Conclusion

This chapter has considered the theme of deprivation in the context of general practice in some detail. It has examined the macro scale of national inequalities in list sizes and the distribution of GPs, and considered the way in which MPA policy has attempted, not without success, to address these inequalities. It has also assessed deprivation on a more local scale by reference to an in-depth study of the omnipresent Jarman index and the deprivation payments system. A description of these issues and policy instruments has been allied with an explanation of the reasons for their shortcomings.

While there are undoubtedly problems with both MPA policy and the deprivation payments system, both represent an important attempt to address a central issue in general practice. Despite their inadequacies, both go some way to ensuring the GPs are available to people in the greatest need and that those GPs are rewarded for practising in what are undeniably difficult settings. Both also have the virtue of simplicity; some might say that they are simplistic, but in the absence of comprehensive, reliable routine data on general practice, and in the light of the independent contractor status of GPs, more sophisticated approaches may yet be some way off.

7

Practice in Context – Urban and Rural General Practice

Boerma *et al.* (1998), in a wide-ranging study of general practice in Europe, noted that the variation in the range of services provided by GPs owes much to the geographical circumstances of the practice location. General practice, like other health services, is more widely available in urban areas. In contrast, the service supply in rural areas can be low, and the concentration of acute services in cities can mean that, in the countryside, GPs are often the only providers of health care. In urban areas, it is often more difficult to regulate access and the use of services. There is often a choice of GPs, and there are plentiful opportunities to access secondary care as an accident and emergency patient. In such circumstances, the traditional gatekeeping role of the GP as the access point to acute care may be reduced. On the other hand, the often-reduced choice of GP and the greater distance from the hospital mean that rural general practices need to provide more comprehensive services.

This chapter pursues these issues in more detail. Its focus is not on the somewhat artificial dichotomy of the rural and the urban. The problematic nature of this distinction is readily acknowledged, particularly in the context of a UK that, outside parts of Scotland, Wales and northern England, is extensively urbanised. Instead, the chapter is concerned with a contrast between general practice in inner cities and in rural areas. The structure of the chapter falls naturally into two parts. In the first, attention focuses on inner city general practice, and in the second, it shifts to rural general practice. In both sections, there is a consideration of the general themes that have emerged in the study of general practice in each type of area and a review of relevant policy measures.

Inner City General Practice

The inner city has long been held to be the locus of particularly marked health problems with studies demonstrating how inner city areas are typified by an above-average concentration of the sick and disabled, as well as populations with characteristics that correlate highly with ill-health, such as unemployment, full-time workers on low pay, single parents, minority ethnic groups, and people living in poor-quality and deteriorating housing conditions (Townsend and Davidson 1988, Acheson 1998). Thus, in Wilkin *et al.* (1987), the inner city Manchester case study area was reported to have a standardised mortality ratio of 122, rising to 137 in deprived parts (1981 data). Data on London from the same time period suggested that, while its inner city demography was not all that unusual, the combination of poor socio-economic circumstances was such that London contained the three worst FPC areas on the Jarman index (Jarman 1989). This distinctiveness has persisted, and it is quintessentially evident that inner cities are difficult environments for the provision of health care, with high concentrations of the type of patient who are known to increase workload.

In addition, inner cities provide conditions in which ill-health can flourish. Mental ill-health is one condition that has often been associated with inner city locations. Lewis *et al.* (1992) report how the prevalence of schizophrenia and rate of first admission to hospital for this disorder are higher in most modern industrialised cities, and in urban compared with rural areas. The incidence of schizophrenia is 1.65 times higher among men brought up in cities than in those who had a rural upbringing, even after taking account of other factors associated with city life. Casey and Tyrer (1990) and Seivewright *et al.* (1991) confirm that psychiatric morbidity is higher in inner city areas and make links with the apparent stresses of urban lifestyles. Other conditions particularly associated with inner city environments include respiratory ill-health linked to high levels of pollution (Bhopal *et al.* 1998).

Finally, inner cities provide poor working conditions and environments in which to practise health care. GPs face not only particularly concentrated levels of patient ill-health and poor socio-economic circumstances, but also higher staff costs, higher land costs and higher property rents. In short, they have to work harder to earn their money. In a *national* health service, there is little or no adaptation to services to take account of the specific conditions prevailing in inner cities. Policies have, as will be seen, been long on problem identification but short on solutions, yet the development of primary health care services in general and GP services in particular is considered to be an important element in combating inner city ill-health.

Inner City GP Service Provision

In the past, attention has often been drawn to the generally inferior structure of primary care services in inner cities, but the evidence for this is equivocal. Much of it is based on the well-documented case of London, where influential and highly publicised reports have made much of a high proportion of elderly and single-handed GPs, as well as a lack of primary care teams working from health centres and a lack of good practice premises (LHPC 1981, DoH 1992c, Turnberg 1998). Other inner cities have been far less well documented and may well be both different and distinct. Even within London, however, paradoxes abound. These range most starkly from the exclusive private general medicine of Harley Street to the low-quality lock-up surgeries of less affluent areas. More generally, London general practice suffers problems of quality at the same time as being officially quantitatively over-doctored (LHPC 1981, Powell 1987).

Outside London, Manchester has been the subject of some attention. Wilkin *et al.* (1987) suggest, on the basis of a population survey and data on GP consultations, that there are relatively few differences between the inner city and more suburban parts of their study area in terms of the use of GP services. They also play down differences in other characteristics, preferring to emphasise the variation between Manchester's and national statistics. Nevertheless, as will be seen below, there are in this study some significant commonalities between Manchester and London in terms of certain key features of practice size and organisation. A complementary study in Manchester confirmed much of Wilkin *et al.*'s conclusions but stressed that there was no evidence of poor-quality general practice in inner city areas (Wood 1983). More recently, a study in Glasgow (Wyke *et al.* 1992) failed to confirm the stereotype of elderly, isolated, single-handed GPs working in deprived areas with a small list size and a lack of resources.

This mention of a stereotype of the inner city GP serves as a useful link to a wider discussion of the possible quantitative and qualitative shortcomings of general practice in inner cities. There are a number of issues that are central to any debate, the first of which concerns the age and ethnic origins of inner city GPs. As has been noted, the inner city is neither a pleasant nor a financially rewarding location in which to practise general medicine. Although certainly challenging (having attracted some dedicated, committed and high-quality practitioners), it also offers workloads that can be heavy and further skewed by the presence of high deprivation. One result of these pressures is that the recruitment of GPs to inner city practices is difficult and, once they have been recruited, turnover tends to be high. In the early years of the NHS, the relative absence of vacancies for GPs meant that this was less of a problem than it is now. At that time, many GPs seized whatever opportunity came along. Later, as general practice grew, vacancies became more plentiful but tended to be where population growth occurred; any inner city vacancies were less popular.

Several consequences flow from this brief history. First, the GPs recruited to inner cities through the 1950s have been retiring over the past 10 years, which has brought a severe recruitment crisis to inner city general practice.

This has had a dual implication. On the one hand, inner city general practice needs to be made more attractive to newly qualified GPs. On the other, its recruitment difficulties mean that other services have had to shoulder an additional burden. Second, the GPs who have retired from inner city practice in recent years had often been practising in the same premises for a number of years. This indicates that the demographic crisis of inner city general practice has been accompanied by a premises crisis. At the time of Knox's (1978) study, for example, 17 per cent of GPs in the East End of Glasgow were over retiring age, and almost half were occupying substandard premises. Finally, the GPs who, in the 1960s and early 1970s, took up inner city opportunities when there were many openings elsewhere are also now retiring. Whether through racism in GP recruitment or personal choice on the part of the GPs themselves, there is considerable evidence that a large proportion of these individuals were GPs who had either been born in or had trained in the Indian subcontinent. For example, in the early 1980s, 40 per cent of the GPs in inner city Manchester had qualified outside the UK (Wilkin *et al.* 1987). It would not be an overstatement to claim that inner city general practice has been substantially dependent on overseas doctors.

A second issue about inner city general practice concerns its relationship to the deprivation status of inner city patients. Here caution must be exercised. Alongside deprivation, many inner cities also possess equal extremes of affluence. Particularly with the advent of inner city gentrification and redevelopment, inner city practices can find themselves balancing the demands of a highly deprived population and the equal but very different demands of an affluent, mobile population. More often, however, the new affluent inner city populations are in a position to pay for private care either in their own right or through their employment. They may also retain a GP elsewhere and are, in any case, less frequent users of general practice.

It is the deprived portion of the inner city population who provide the most workload for inner city GPs, yet the characteristics of the deprived population are also those which tend to indicate a lower likelihood of compliance with preventive health measures and less interest in health promotion. This means that inner city GPs are less likely to benefit from target payment systems or health promotion payments. Potential recruits to inner city general practice may thus be dissuaded from applying for posts in deprived areas because of the heavy workload and poorer financial remuneration. Social deprivation certainly has a real effect on primary care working patterns. Consultation rates are higher and consultation times shorter and, within each crowded consultation, patients with multiple problems create a heavy workload (Watt 1996).

The third issue concerning general practice is perhaps the one that receives the most attention in the literature. Chapter 1 charted the gradual disappearance of the single-handed GP. Yet, against this picture, single-handed general practice remains very much a feature of urban, particularly inner city, health care. Wilkin *et al.* (1987), for example, found nearly double the national average of single-handed practices in their case study area and nearly half the national average of practices with five or more partners. Jarman (1981) reports figures of three times and one-third for the same indicators in London. Fry (1983) referred to this formerly very common way of working as 'a cause for concern'. The reasons for this view can be found in a presumption that a large practice is now the norm and working alone is synonymous with having poor premises, being infrequently available out of hours and having little integration with the primary health care team (Morley *et al.* 1981). To this list could be added, from a GP's viewpoint, the difficulty in having any break from work without recourse to costly locum or deputising services and the difficulty of ensuring an adequate income stream in the face of an inevitable inability to offer the extra services provided for under the 1990 GP contract. Tudor Hart (1988) affirms this picture in his recollections of his own early years as a single-handed GP in Inner London in shop-front premises with poor equipment and unpleasant working conditions.

Green (1993, 1996) provides perhaps the most comprehensive analysis of single-handed general practice. She confirms the view that it has long been assumed that single-handed general practice is dying out as a form of service provision, but notes that some 20 per cent of GPs in Lambeth, Southwark and Lewisham were practising on their own in 1992. These GPs were more likely to have registered before 1960, to have qualified outside Britain and not to undertake health promotion clinics or employ a practice nurse. They were, in short, old fashioned. Yet, as Green rightly and sensitively notes, this characterisation cuts both ways. Many single-handed inner city GPs saw themselves as the last bastion of individualism and personal control in an increasingly impersonal, 'modern' service. They claimed to stand for continuity of care and courtesy, and viewed the reforms to general practice as a threat to their more traditional style. For some, single-handed general practice was a matter of definite choice, and lists were kept low to enable a close familiarity with patients. This analysis resonates with Curtis's (1987) claim that, for some people in the East End of London, the single-handed GP remains a well-liked figure with whom there exists rapport and trust – in short, a genuine 'family doctor'.

Two further points can be made about single-handed general practice. Armstrong (1985) and Horrobin and McIntosh (1983) provide a reminder that, although it may be more prevalent in the inner city, it is by no means a vestigial presence only in inner city areas. The single-handed GP is also a feature of more remote rural areas. These authors suggest that, in both the inner city and deep rural areas, there is a sense in which the environment aids the continued survival of single-handed general practice. The lone GP serves a precise and well-defined community; he (less often she) is a community figure with an organic relationship not only to his or her patients, but also to the wider locale. This analysis would suggest that, as traditional communities break down, so traditional ways of delivering general practice become eroded. The commodification, modernisation and even industrialisation of general practice is thus a process that goes hand in hand with the changing relationship of the GP to the community. This sociological perspective is, however, matched by another more empirically grounded point. It is inappropriate to see single-handed general practice as a uniformly undifferentiated category. Instead, it can take a number of forms. There are relatively few genuinely 'lone' single-handed practitioners on call 24 hours a day all year round. Most use deputising services or participate in cooperatives to cover off-call periods. Many also work regularly alongside another single-handed practice, providing mutual cover and a partnership in all but name (Wilkin *et al.* 1987). Finally, despite stories of practices based in lock-up shops, a number work from health centres and share in the communally provided services of such facilities.

List size in inner city general practice is another issue that receives a great deal of attention. It is generally lower in inner city areas, although the evidence is again varied. Wilkin *et al.* (1987) found that the smallest per capita lists were in two-person partnership practices. They noted, however, that, other than with single-handed GPs, there is a great deal of difficulty in providing a realistic estimate of the impact of list size on care as practices habitually pool their lists. Evidence for the review of primary health care in Inner London suggested that some GPs chose to maintain low lists to enhance a closeness to their patients or reduce the stresses of providing care to high-demand patients, but others did so for financial reasons in that a low but NHS-funded list provided a buffer for the development of a private practice (LHPC 1981). Wilkin *et al.* (1987), in contrast, found no evidence that list sizes were artificially or deliberately held down in inner city Manchester. Indeed, they noted that over half of the lowest lists in their case study areas were in deprived areas of declining population where the GPs must have been struggling to ensure the financial viability of their practices. They also found no evidence to suggest that having fewer patients meant that a GP was able to devote more time to a list and see more patients or offer longer consultation times.

One inevitable implication of low list size in inner cities is that more GPs are required to serve the population, and it is unlikely that the area will fulfil the criterion for designation as under-doctored. This limits the turnover of GPs and contributes to the demographic problem alluded to above. A decision to have a low list size can also mean that GPs may be selective about taking people onto their lists and be more likely to remove difficult patients. This can in turn have two consequences: patient choice is reduced, and there is a greater pressure on alternative forms of first-line care, most notably, as will be seen below, on the accident and emergency departments of acute hospitals.

Geographical Issues and Inner City General Practice

To the extent that they vary within and between inner cities, and between inner cities and other areas, the issues discussed so far in this section all raise questions concerning the geography of general practice. There are, however, two issues that are of particular relevance to the development of a geography of general practice in inner cities. The first of these concerns the areas served by inner city general practices. Any general practice, whether urban or rural, will have a majority of its patient list living close to the surgery, and the number of registered patients will fall off with distance from the practice.

Overlying this general 'distance decay' are a multiplicity of factors that determine which practice gains the registration of a particular individual patient. In urban areas, this tends to lead to very diffuse patient registration fields, or 'catchment areas'. Nonetheless, under the 1990 GP contract, GPs are obliged to define their catchment area. Jenkins and Campbell (1996) relate the size of general practice catchment areas in one London borough to list size, deprivation payments, medical staffing and locally and nationally recognised measures of quality. Catchment area size varied greatly between practices, showing an almost 150-fold difference between the largest and the smallest practices. Substantial differences also existed between practices in each of four locally assigned quality bands. The weakest practices had catchment areas three times as large as those of the strongest practices. A calculated measure of patient dispersion showed that the practice population of the strongest practices was four times as densely clustered as that of the weakest practices, whose patients were more widely geographically dispersed. This finding suggests that practices with lists that are relatively concentrated in spatial terms are likely to be of higher quality.

A second geographical theme concerns the venue from which general medical care is provided. The provision of GP care is a matter not just of how much there is and the quality of that care. It is also about where it is provided. Those who have to travel further to a GP are disadvantaged. The evidence suggests that patients who live close to a surgery consult up to a third more often than those living more than 3.5 km away (Whitehouse 1985). While such spatial inaccessibility is seldom a major issue in inner cities, it is complicated by opportunity factors that can have a specific inner city dimension. Thus the opening hours of single-handed practices may limit access opportunity. Similarly, deprived populations dependent on public transport may effectively have less opportunity for access. Knox (1978) provided a classic study on this theme. Using data from Aberdeen, Edinburgh, Glasgow and Dundee, he found spatial access to be inversely related to socio-economic status, to the extent that inner city general practice suffered a triple penalty with social deprivation, qualitative inadequacies in practice provision and spatial disadvantage. As well as inner cities, Knox suggested that peripheral local authority housing estates and rural areas were also similarly disadvantaged. Jones and Kirby (1982), working in Reading, confirmed the salient features of this analysis: three types of area typically have cumulative spatial inaccessibility to GP services. High-status affluent areas are perhaps the least problematic. Residents have private transport and prefer to travel rather than accept the potential intrusion and traffic problems associated with a (usually) large general practice facility. Elderly residents in such areas may, however, experience some problems. New owner-occupied estates are a second spatially disadvantaged area. These areas suffer facility lag as general practice (and MPA designations) adjust to acknowledge new opportunities. They are, however, attractive areas in which to practise and are at some stage likely to draw in an appropriate level of provision. The third sort of spatially disadvantaged area is more problematic. Areas of substantial public or social housing are unattractive to GPs, and house residents are unable to pay for travel.

To an extent, the issue of spatial access to health care is exacerbated by the growth in multipartner practices, particularly health centres, and the decline of the single-handed GP. Eckstein (1958) reports how, in the first 10 years of the NHS, only a handful of health centres were opened despite the health centre being seen as the future of primary care. Between 1960 and 1973, however, the number of health centres rose from 18 to 468 (Ottewill and Wall 1990). This growth inevitably entailed the movement of existing GPs into more centralised premises. Jones and Moon (1987) trace the impact of this process on one suburban local authority housing estate, noting how people who were once close to a small practice became relatively distant from the new health centre. This simple spatial distancing also hides a deeper sociological process. For Armstrong (1985), the rise of the health centre can be seen as a modernist project separating home and work for the GP. The abandonment of the parlour surgery, where the GP's work and home were literally in the same place, for the health centre saw the GP separate home from work metaphorically as well as physically. By breaching a personal tie to an area, the growth of health centres contributed to the decline of the GP as a community figure.

Inner City General Practice Utilisation

Given the association of deprivation, workload and health service usage noted in the previous chapter, it will not be surprising that there are strong inner city dimensions to GP service usage. Carr-Hill and colleagues (1996), in their multilevel analysis of national variations in the GP consultation rate, found that factors associated with urban locations were most strongly associated with a higher consultation rate. Indeed, among their significant factors was a dummy variable indicating residence in an urban area. Bowling *et al.* (1991) indicated that the utilisation of health and social services was found to be higher in the urban area, increasing with age. Li and Taylor (1991) compare the immunisation uptake rate in general practice surgeries and community child health clinics in four health districts of North East Thames Regional Health Authority. Children resident in rural and suburban areas had a greater uptake than those in inner cities , the odds ratios for not being fully immunised being 3.0 times greater among children resident in inner cities than among those in rural and suburban districts. Griffiths *et al.* (1997), in a study of asthma morbidity in the East End of London, found that a higher admission rate for diagnoses of asthma was most strongly associated with a small size of practice partnership; the admission rates of single-handed and two-partner practices were higher than those of practices with three or more principals by 1.7 times and 1.3 times respectively. This association was independent of prescribing behaviour, measures of practice resources and the characteristics of practice populations. Finally, Leese and Bosanquet (1995) found that a minority of practices (27 per cent) in the London inner city area achieved the higher target level for cervical smear testing, compared with 88 per cent for London as a whole. A similar trend was apparent for childhood immunisation.

Wilkin *et al.* (1987) yet again provide a useful antidote to extreme perspectives on the concentration of high GP service usage in deprived parts of inner cities. Figure 7.1 offers a graphical portrayal of their data on GP consultations. It is evident that, on the one hand, variations between different parts of the city are relatively slight. The figure does, however, also indicate that the consultation rate is higher in deprived areas in comparison to affluent areas although not to any great extent different between the inner and outer city.

There are, of course, a number of specific problems associated with GP service usage in inner urban areas. Wood *et al.* (1997) provide sound documentation of the difficulties of delivering health care to homeless people. Many studies have indicated the health status of homeless people to be typically poorer than that of the general population, various studies indicating a high prevalence of psychiatric illness, drug or alcohol misuse and associated socio-medical problems. Only 55 per cent of inner city practices in their study would contemplate fully registering a homeless person. While this figure is higher than in other areas, it indicates something of the problems facing homeless people seeking general medical care in inner cities. It results from the perceived difficulties of providing care to homeless people as well as, perhaps more crucially, the possible adverse effects of homeless people on GP contract targets. Herity *et al.* (1997) raise a further issue. Although their study

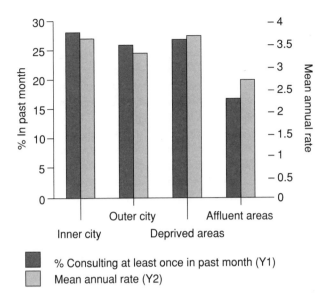

Figure 7.1   GP consultations in Manchester, mid-1980s

was based in the Republic of Ireland, it has wider implications. In an attempt to track individuals for a screening programme in an inner city area, the response following two invitations was only 20 per cent. Over 20 per cent of addresses were incorrect – the difficulties of delivering care to a highly mobile population compound the problems of a high need population.

If people are falling through the net of general practice, it is evident that they are seeking primary health care elsewhere, if indeed they seek care at all. The established view is that, for those who do seek care, the key alternative to the GP is the hospital accident and emergency department. Ward *et al.* (1996), in a study of St Mary's Hospital, Paddington, accident and emergency department, found that 16.6 per cent of accident and emergency attenders during their study period were suitable for primary care. McKee *et al.* (1990) suggested that distance from an accident and emergency department was an important factor in the rate of attendance, but neither the socio-economic status of the attender's area of residence nor the characteristics of the general practice were significant factors in explaining attendance. It is this substitution of accident and emergency for GP care that has been most remarked upon in the policy studies of Inner London general practice that provide the subject matter for much of the next section.

General Practice in Inner London

Notwithstanding the conclusion of Wilkin *et al.* (1987) that London is different, there is a wealth of documentation and policy prescription on general practice in London. This therefore provides an appropriate case study. Benzeval *et al.* (1991) provide a good overview of the history of London's health problems and the various attempts to address these difficulties. They show in particular how these problems were exacerbated by the workings of the NHS funding formula designed to pursue equity in funding across the regions (DHSS 1976b) and its various successors, most notably the internal market. The funding formulae and the internal market both moved resources away from London and initiated pressure for the rationalisation of acute care.

Alongside this pressure ran a realisation that primary care was also in need of major surgery if it was ever to provide the basis for a primary care-led NHS in the capital. Besides poor socio-economic conditions, poor standardised mortality rates, a high population mobility (30–40 per cent annually in some parts of the city), a high proportion of people without English as a first language, and substantial levels of homelessness, substance abuse and poverty, there was a high proportion of GPs not in group practice and a substantial number aged over 65. There were also large variations in the distribution of GPs within Inner London as well as between Inner and Outer London (Benzeval and Judge 1996).

Primary health care in Inner London

The 1981 report of the working group on primary health care in Inner London (LHPC 1981) serves as a useful starting point for discussion. At the time of publication it tended to be referred to as the Acheson Report in honour of its chair, Sir Donald Acheson, later to be Chief Medical Officer, but the subsequent blossoming of Acheson Reports has lessened the utility of this naming. Four themes can be singled out in the LHPC (1981): list size, registration, GP availability and practice size, and the age structure of general practice.

With regard to list size, the report showed a marked concern related to GPs with a small list. It was suggested that GPs can have few patients compared with their colleagues for a variety of reasons. They may be starting out, they may work on their own and restrict their list in order to ensure that they have time to deal personally with patients and reduce their reliance on deputising services, or they may deliberately restrict their list so that they can operate a private practice. The report laid great stress on the last suggestion: that some GPs were deliberately limiting the size of their NHS list so that they could draw on NHS resources to underpin their provision to private patients with a guaranteed income stream. In short, it hinted that private practice was riding on the back of NHS base funding. The evidence for this allegation was slight, and it is perhaps best to view it as a hypothesis rather than a sustained, evidence-based conclusion. Certainly, as reported above, Wilkin *et al.* (1987) did not find substantiating evidence for this in their study in Manchester.

A second issue of concern was registration. The report suggested that up to 30 per cent of the population of some inner city districts might not be registered with a GP. Substitute coverage was provided by deputising services, which often responded to all calls rather than only those that they were forwarded, and by extensive use of accident and emergency departments. Reasons for non-registration with GPs were acknowledged to be complex. Important factors included the high mobility of the London population and delayed registrations by new arrivals in the city, putting off registration until sick. It was recognised that the gap between the size of the London population and the number registered with GPs was, to some extent, a reflection of the significant number of residents maintaining a second address in London but registered elsewhere. It was also appreciated that homeless people might try to register and fail, and that minority ethnic groups might not have been afforded appropriate information on how to register. Finally, it was suggested that some non-registering people simply did not wish to register. Evidence was cited of people who had tried several GPs before getting registered and who had been refused by their nearest practice.

Once registered, the report held, appropriately enough, that full GP services should be available, but the reality of this core NHS commitment was far less satisfactory. Particular difficulties were found to exist outside standard 'office hours', and, in a related study, it was calculated that some 20 per cent of out-of-hours calls resulted in the patient resorting to hospital care (Richards *et al.* 1981). Almost half of the Inner London practices contacted during the study were found not to be contactable during the day, the greatest difficulty being posed by single-handed practices. GP availability was thus seen as intimately connected with issues surrounding practice size. Small practices were felt to militate against the teamwork necessary to provide round-the-clock care. They were also associated with a greater propensity to use accident and emergency care as a substitute for GP care. Accordingly, group practice (defined as a partnership of more than three GPs) was very strongly encouraged.

The relatively low level of group practice – 60 per cent of Inner London practices at the time not having more than three partners compared with a national mean of 30 per cent (LHPC 1981) – was also discussed in terms of the fourth key concern of the report: the age profile of GPs in Inner London. It was suggested that older GPs were less attracted by group practice, and were simultaneously both more individualistic yet more set in their ways and untrained for the compromises inherent in partnership working. In a substudy of GPs over retirement age, it was also found that many carried on simply out of intense dedication and enjoyment, although, for over half, finance was also important as many had, even over a lifetime's service to the NHS, not accrued adequate pension contributions.

The prescriptions of the report on primary care in Inner London (LHPC 1981) were essentially those of the Royal Commission on the NHS (1979). The report recommended more health centres, the introduction of salaried GPs and a reduced list size. In the event, a combination of a small degree of protectionism on the part of a minority of GPs and a large absence of adequate funding from an unsympathetic government, as well as from health authorities facing penalties for excess funding to London and high financial demands from acute services, ensured that the sole real impact of the report was an extra £9m over four years for grants to improve practice premises in inner city areas and additional support for the training of health visitors.

The inquiry into London's health service

LHPC (1981) contained a focused analysis of primary care in Inner London. The second report to be considered in this subsection had primary care as an objective but was substantially more concerned with acute services. The Tomlinson Review of London's health service (DoH 1992c) was preceded by an independent study conducted by the King's Fund (1992) and followed by two further significant reports, the governmental response to Tomlinson (DoH 1993) and a coda to the review process (Turnberg 1998). Together, the suite of studies constituted a comprehensive analysis of the crisis of acute care precipitated by the cumulative effects of the regional funding redirection mentioned above and the impact of the internal market NHS reforms of the early 1990s.

What faced London acute care was, in essence, a situation of too many hospital beds. Maxwell (1993) provides a reminder that London was not, however, the only UK city facing such a situation. Baggott (1994) claims that London in the early 1990s had some 25 per cent more beds than the national average. This situation had developed in response to historical contingencies and the capital's position as an international centre of excellence for medical education. This overprovision of acute beds, albeit disputed (Jarman 1993), was, and remains, accompanied by high staff costs, a high staff turnover and inpatient stays that are longer than average. This situation had been sustained for many years but became untenable as the internal market began to bite and non-London health authorities began to question the financial sense of referring patients to costly London hospitals, seeking to fund provision outside the capital. London NHS hospital trusts were faced with a diminishing demand for their services, while, at the same time, London health authorities were seeking to respond to the agenda set by the review of primary health care and develop better quality primary care.

Not surprisingly, the prescription provided by Tomlinson was one of the rationalisation of acute care. Equally unsurprisingly, an important subtext was the need to redirect resources towards primary health care. This was in part a recognition that, despite a decade since the publication of the review of primary health care (LHPC 1981), primary health care in Inner London still faced many of the problems identified in the earlier report. Thus, even by local definitions, fewer than 50 per cent of premises in London met acceptable minimum standards, nearly all practice premises in the rest of England being above minimum standard. The proportion of GPs aged over 65 was still some 30 per cent above the national average, the proportion of single-handed practices remained at over twice the national level, and recruitment continued to be problematic (DoH 1992c). These problems were held to have resulted in a poor achievement of contractual targets and a tendency to concentrate only on the basic elements of general practice (Boyle and Smaje 1992). The crux of the linkage of primary to acute care was a claim that better primary care might reduce the use of accident and emergency departments for general medical care and shorten hospital stay. London patients, it was argued, stayed in hospital longer because of poor local primary care.

The Conservative government largely accepted Tomlinson's diagnosis and initiated a programme to pump-prime primary care initiatives (DoH 1993). The London Initiative Zone (LIZ) programme was established to facilitate an improvement in the standard of primary care in London. LIZ investment had three components: service development, continuing medical education incentives to encourage the recruitment and retention of inner city GPs, and the introduction of flexibilities in workforce regulations to support small practices (Turnberg 1998). The latter development was of particular significance in that it sought to aid single-handed practices in skills development and also allowed for the employment of GP assistants. Investment in LIZ was predicted to amount to some £402.9m by the end of 1998/99. Of this, over £100m was spent on improving premises and a further £20m on increasing the numbers of GP practice staff.

By the time of the Turnberg Report (Turnberg 1998), essentially a New Labour ratification of much of the Tomlinson Report save for the contentious reprieve of the St Bartholemew's Hospital West Smithfield site, the LIZ processes were largely complete. They had also been overtaken by the evolving role of GPs in health care commissioning (see Chapter 4) and other measures, including an increased willingness to countenance forms of GP employment other than the traditional one of an independent contractor. Thus, on the one hand, there was pressure for the LIZ measures to be extended and the number of GPs practising in London to be increased proportionally to match the rest of the country. The adjustments to MPA policy (see Chapter 6) to ensure 'really equitable distribution' were commended, and extensions to the LIZ workforce flexibilities were suggested to permit the easier employment of salaried GPs and enhanced reward systems for Inner London GP principals. On the other hand, it was noted that GP commissioning in its various forms had helped to reduce the isolation of GPs, particularly single-handed practitioners, and had improved access to support services. Furthermore, it was argued that peer group pressure was an inevitable concomitant of the new enhanced role of the GP and that this would help to raise average standards, as well as ensure a full and effective coverage of resident populations, including populations otherwise marginalised or excluded from GP care.

Rural General Practice

As the RCGP (1998) argues, paradoxically, in its fact sheet on inner city general practice:

> poverty and deprivation are not confined to the geographical inner city areas... It must be recognised that there is certainly an excess of disadvantage in the geographical inner city, despite islands of renewal created by gentrification schemes, but post industrial semi-rural areas such as the Welsh valleys and post-war housing estates on the edge of towns share many features of 'inner city' deprivation.

In this section, attention extends beyond the 'semi-rural' to encompass a consideration of general practice in remoter rural areas. The intention is to reveal both commonalities and points of difference in terms of the delivery of GP care in an environment that, in comparison to the inner city, has received far less attention (Cox 1995).

Before commencing this examination, a brief word on rural health status is in order. On the matter of comparative health status, the differences between urban and rural areas are complex. Phillimore and Reading (1992) confirm that rural health inequalities have been neglected and suggest, on the basis of an extensive study of northern England, that, although inequalities in urban areas are, in a general sense, wider than those in rural areas in so far as the gap between the worst and the best is larger, there are parts of the rural north of England that return levels of health status which are, by any analysis, poor. On the basis of matching urban and rural areas for comparable levels of socio-economic status, it is clear that poorer areas in either environment tend to have similar levels of health. Remote rural areas that are not markedly impoverished do, however, have a significant advantage in terms of health status.

Reading *et al.* (1993) offer a confirmation that ill-health is not confined to urban areas but confirm that a more substantial disadvantage is conferred by urban residence. They go on, however, to recognise, as do Shucksmith *et al.*

(1996) and the Joseph Rowntree Foundation (1994), that ill-health in rural areas is the subject of marked stratification. Thus, 25 per cent of rural households live in 'absolute poverty' (Bradley 1987) and, in remote areas such as the Outer Hebrides, almost the whole population are on 'poverty' incomes (Cox 1998). Ill-health is concentrated in traditional rural populations, notably in the ageing rural working class – 35 per cent of poor rural households are elderly people living alone. Newer rural populations, such as commuters, second-home owners and even retirees, are relatively more healthy. Rural areas are therefore diverse but in a different way from cities, and the juxtaposition of the old and the new rural populations can mean that an affluent landowner and a socially isolated, underprivileged tenant landworker may be each other's closest neighbour.

Rural GP Service Provision

Rural health care provision is a significant area of study in many countries, but this is not the case in the UK. Arguably the best available evidence on the delivery of GP services in rural areas in the UK remains that of Cartwright and Anderson (1981). This work suggested that rural GPs have a smaller list size and make more hospital referrals. It also indicated that rural GPs were more likely than urban GPs to undertake work themselves rather than in collaboration with a wider team, and were also more likely to undertake more work and receive fewer 'trivial' consultations. Their analysis suggested that the rate of home visiting was no greater in rural areas. While this is clearly a very brief summary of a substantial study and refers to a situation that is now somewhat distant in time, it should be clear that there appear to be recognisable elements of traditionalism in the portrayal of rural general practice. The suggestion was one of practitioners who 'go further' with their patients and may work in more traditional ways, in terms of both a lower affinity for teamwork and a greater propensity to refer for hospital care.

General practice in rural areas, however, also faces a problem that is, to a large extent, a distinctly rural matter. Although it could be argued that single-handed urban GPs are in some ways isolated from the stimulus of partnership, they are not isolated by distance in the same as their rural colleagues can be. The impact of isolation can work in two ways. Keeping personal development in group practices going when the distance between practices and local centres of continuing education is large is not easy. When a practice is both rural and single-handed, the difficulties are compounded (Cox 1995). The difficulty of sustaining personal development, satisfying continuing education requirements, and even achieving necessary rest and recovery, are particularly complicated by the problems entailed in sustaining out-of-hours and locum cover in remote rural areas where, for example, potential partners for cooperative cover schemes may be too distant to be an effective substitute for out-of-hours calls and deputising services may be based only in larger towns.

The second impact of isolation on rural general practice lies in its relationship to the physical accessibility of GP services. Despite rural population growth and a consequent increase in the size of many villages, service provision in rural areas has diminished (Shucksmith 1996). General practice has not been immune from this pressure and has tended to concentrate in larger settlements (RDC 1998). Only 17 per cent of rural parishes in England have a permanent general practice in the parish. Geographically, the better provided rural parishes tend to be in the south and south-west. At least partially as a consequence, consultation rates tend to be lower in more remote rural parishes. An allied development has been the reduction in rural public transport. People without their own transport and those with mobility problems have increasing difficulty in gaining access to services, and independent transport is often an expensive necessity.

Largely as a consequence of extensive work at the University of East Anglia, the accessibility of health services is one theme in rural health care that has received significant attention. The provision of branch surgeries has been a particular focus. Fearn (1983) found that branch surgeries in Norfolk were provided in pubs, converted barns, GP's homes and village halls, only some 20 per cent being purpose built. Branch opening hours varied but were not extensive. Three hours for one or two days each week was typical. Branch surgeries essentially provided services to the local poor, those without access to cars and elderly people (Fearn *et al.* 1984), thus enhancing access to primary medical care. They are, however, expensive to run, and as a consequence have been decreasing in number over many years.

Bentham and Haynes (1992) evaluate one attempt to provide a cost-effective alternative. They consider the use of a caravan as a general practice mobile branch surgery in rural Norfolk. The consultation rates marginally increased during the first year that the caravan surgery was provided as a replacement service in a village where there had previously been a conventional branch surgery. In contrast, in a village where the mobile surgery was a new facility, there was a substantial increase in consultation. Bentham and Haynes suggested that the service reduced the problems of physical access in remote villages to the level of those villages where a main surgery is situated. Such innovations apart, however, the level of GP service provision in more remote rural areas remains low. Jones *et al.* (1998), albeit in a consideration of the particular case of asthma patients, show how, after controlling for relevant factors, rural residents are three times less likely to have ever visited a GP if they live outside a settlement containing a surgery, and the likelihood of consultation declines with distance from a surgery.

It should at this point be briefly noted that other alternatives to the provision of branch surgeries include nurse care, in the form of either outreach by the primary care team or nurse-triaged telephone consultation schemes. The emergence of NHS Direct as a possible first point of access to medical care offers much to more remote rural areas, although it demands a comprehensive evaluation. Evidence from studies of telemedicine schemes to date (Harrison *et al.* 1997) suggests that GP and patient acceptance is high. Armstrong and Haston (1997) report on a telemedicine link between the accident and emergency department of a remote community hospital and that of a large urban hospital. Results indicated that both the GPs running the community hospital and the accident and emergency consultants felt that teleconsultation had improved patient care. The link avoided the transfer of 70 patients and saved some £65,000 over the study period. More evidence of this nature is, however, required before it can conclusively be claimed that rural inaccessibility to health care can be safely, effectively and efficiently addressed by telemedicine.

Why does the physical inaccessibility of GP care in more remote rural areas matter? The treatment of acute myocardial infarction among the residents of such areas provides a sound answer to this question. Rawles *et al.* (1998) compared city, suburban and country practices referring patients to a single district general hospital in north-east Scotland. GPs were the first medical contact in 97 per cent of calls by rural residents. This figure compares with that of 68 per cent for city and suburban patients. One-third of the rural patients went on to receive treatment from their GPs, 93 per cent of these patients being treated within the national standard 'call-to-needle' time of 90 minutes. Murphy *et al.* (1996) found relatively little difference between urban and rural GPs in terms of response times for acute myocardial infarctions: 10 and 15 minutes respectively. If, however, the rural GP did not treat but referred the patient on to hospital, the call-to-needle time increased significantly, to an average of 40 minutes for rural patients. This delay time suggests that, in order to meet current guidelines, initial treatment by GPs is generally essential in rural areas. The role of the rural GP in the management of patients with suspected acute myocardial infarction is thus important both quantitatively and in terms of enhancing survival.

Policy and the Rural GP

There are two main ways in which health care policy attempts to address the problems of general practice in rural areas. The first concerns enhanced payments to GPs practising in rural areas. As part of the 1990 contract, rural practice payments were revised. The basic practice allowance was enhanced for patients living in sparsely populated areas. There was a recognition that 'rural practice makes particular demands because of the greater area to be covered and the limit on the size of lists' (GB Departments of Health 1989:9). A new rural supplement became payable in respect of the number of patients living in electoral wards with a population below a set threshold. It suffers problems very similar to those outlined with respect to deprivation payments (see Chapter 6). Single-handed GPs practising in very isolated areas (isolated GPs) were recognised as being at a particular disadvantage in so far as they were acknowledged to have difficulty getting away from the practice at any time let alone for vacations, and might also be socially and professionally isolated, missing out on vocational education opportunities. An associates allowance was proposed and envisaged as a scheme primarily for Scotland. It enabled the employment of an associate GP who might be shared with a number of similar practices in order to provide cover for time off and vacations.

The second policy adjustment relevant to rural general practice is the provision for GPs to dispense drugs. In urban areas, this function is almost always undertaken by community pharmacists. For a GP, having dispensing status involves distance from the chemist or serious difficulty in reaching the chemist. These two ways of attaining dispensing status generally amount to the same thing. The actual government regulations (the NHS Pharmaceutical Regulations 1992) allow GPs to dispense for patients who live in rural areas more than one mile from a pharmacy. In 1994, there were an estimated 4,636 dispensing doctors (14 per cent of the total number of GPs) in the UK, covering approximately eight million people (14 per cent of the population). This is a rise of 30 per cent since 1984. In the UK, approximately 94 per cent of prescriptions are dispensed by chemists, but the number of items dispensed by doctors has increased by more than 4 per cent each year for the past decade compared with some 3 per cent growth in dispensed prescriptions by community pharmacists (OHE 1995).

Dispensing status is, for many rural GPs, more than just a nice little earner. It has been recognised (Cox 1995) as an important financial buffer for many rural GPs as it provides a practice with an additional income stream. It is needed to bolster rural GP incomes in the face of low list size and low opportunities for other forms of care activity, such as private practice. It is also under threat from a number of quarters. The extended role of the community pharmacist is perhaps the most significant challenge. This sees pharmacists providing a certain level of health care advice alongside their prescribing duties (Hassell *et al.* 1996, 1997). It has led pharmacists to expand their practices, and they can do this with lower overheads than GPs, for example by opening branch pharmacies in village stores. There are also, at the time of writing, proposals to amend the one mile rule to two miles, at least in Northern Ireland. Against these threats it must, however, be noted that, on the limited available evidence, prescribing by rural GPs is relatively cost-efficient. Stewart-Brown *et al.* (1995) suggest that the continuing rise in prescribing costs has been least marked among dispensing fundholders, and Pringle and Morton-Jones (1994) report that semi-rural areas have a low number of high-cost items per patient.

Conclusion

This chapter began by stating the foolishness of a distinction between rural and urban health care. There are clearly many issues in common between both areas. Some issues have become synonymous with one or other type of area: single-handed practices with inner urban areas, problems of accessibility with rural areas. Yet these are seldom completely specific to a particular type of area, and there are also important contextual differences between rural and urban areas in terms of the practice of general practice. Problem diagnosis has been strong in the inner city, although less well documented in rural areas. Policy developments such as rural payments, the LIZ provisions and dispensing status have a certain spatial specificity. Pringle and Heath (1997) are perhaps right in their suggestion that a more considered policy response would be one that implemented different contracts for different locations, contracts that would reflect the state of general practice in a particular area as well as need, and make allowance for the costs of practice in areas with high land prices and high employment costs or which are remote. This would, however, go against the principle of the single national contract that currently underpins general practice throughout the UK.

8

GPs and their Patients – Relationships Defined by Profession and Policy

It is an inescapable fact that the primary dynamic in general practice, the clinical or therapeutic doctor–patient relationship, has been increasingly conditioned by extraneous factors. Government policy and the views of an increasingly sophisticated 'clientele' reflect a growing scepticism with the coercive potency of a professional code that presumes that, left to their own devices, doctors will do their best for their patient. Thereafter, government interests diverge from those of the atomised individual, more recent policy agendas emphasising responsibility for resource management and for the health care of local populations. In this chapter, the attempts by government to create a more consumer-conscious service will be evaluated, as will profession-sponsored initiatives, such as practice participation groups. The complaints process and the increase in litigation will be discussed, not merely in the context of failed professional–client relationships, but also as trends indicative of the gulf between raised patient expectations and the ability of GPs, as resource allocators, to meet them. The impact of these and other emerging pressures, such as the tension between the GP's responsibility to her or his individual patient and that of the practice or locality population, will be explored.

Traditional accounts of professional–client relationships, including medicine, emphasise the obligation of the professional to promote the interests of the client. It is a concept that has been perhaps more vigorously promulgated by medicine both to justify clinical freedom and to reassure the client (Freidson 1970a), who in matters of health is more vulnerable than in other life challenges. While the practice of medicine may be an art involving communication with its public, it is essentially embedded in science. In order to succeed in the task of deciphering the complexities of the human body, medicine has reduced it to a complex set of interrelated biochemical systems, cells and genetic material. Historically, this biomedical model of medical science has dominated the practice of medicine, emphasising pathologies and depersonalising the patient (Jewson 1976). The technological intricacy of medicine, its reductionist approach and a lack of sophistication in the general public indulged consultation styles that have been described as paternalistic and directive in nature, maintaining a high degree of control over the consultation and its outcome. The responsibility does not always lie with the doctor: there is also evidence indicating that some patients have preferred to surrender responsibility for decision-making to their doctor, thus reflecting a passive consumerist style (Lloyd *et al.* 1991).

More recent approaches in medicine, particularly evident in general practice literature, have emphasised the importance of social and environmental contexts to health. The consultation, combined with an holistic, patient-centred approach, is seen as the locus of the therapeutic process. There may, however, be dissonance between expressed theory and practice. May *et al.* (1996) found that while some GPs embraced this model of consultation, controls were exercised to manage not only time, but also the subject matter raised in the consultation. Beyond this, evidence is difficult to find on the proportion of GPs who practise patient-centred consultations, or on their level of consistency. While it would be too crude and instrumentalist an analysis to suggest that health policies impact on different practice styles in different ways, it may well be that those practitioners who have a more open and less paternalistic approach to patients will find that relationships are better able to withstand the challenges to come as GPs become increasingly involved in decisions concerning resource allocation.

Since today's medical practitioners rarely contract directly with clients to provide a service, it is axiomatic to the principle of clinical autonomy that third parties, the state and insurers of health care, do not interfere in clinical decision-making. Past attempts to preserve clinical autonomy have served the medical profession as much as they have aimed to secure appropriate treatment for the patient with minimal regard for the cost. Doctors in industrialised democracies have experienced good levels of income, control over their sphere of work and considerable influence in determining health policy. In the UK, in comparison with the severe constraints imposed by the friendly societies in the late nineteenth and early twentieth centuries, state-subsidised general practice has enjoyed considerable managerial and clinical autonomy. This has been reinforced by the longevity of tenure of most GPs and, not infrequently, their investment in practice premises. The 'ownership' of general practice, in the literal as well as the metaphorical sense, has placed GPs in a more ambiguous position than most doctors within the NHS and strengthened their claims for managerial independence.

In the UK, as elsewhere, the state has intervened in the domain of medical practice. Since the mid-1980s, measures introduced to general practice and the wider NHS have required GPs to consider both the efficacy and the cost of treatment. Pressure in the health care field has required GPs increasingly to advocate for patients, as well as justify their own clinical activities. (Further reference to clinical governance is made in Chapter 5.) Despite early rumblings of opposition to such measures as the limited prescribing list, the message appears to have been driven home. A survey on core professional values conducted by the BMA (1995b), in which GPs were the largest group responding, found that 98.6 per cent of doctors felt that clinical freedom was important but that doctors also had an obligation to use resources effectively. A recognition of the need for treatment effectiveness against a background of finite resources inevitably places an obligation on GPs to consider the collective needs of their list patients and beyond rather than their traditional view idealising individual needs.

Doctor–patient relationships are defined by contractual as well as economic and professional considerations. These were in the past combined in an arrangement whereby the private patient paid a fee directly to the doctor, but the creation of the NHS led to a reduction in the amount of private general practice. The state sets out the terms of service and contracts with GPs, but attention to and monitoring of the GP's performance only began in a meaningful way after the implementation of the 1990 GP contract. Thus, for many years in the NHS, the combination of professional ethic and mild surveillance by the FPCs (FHSAs after 1990 and health authorities after April 1996) was deemed sufficient to maintain non-clinical standards of professional practice.

The new contract (see Chapters 3 and 5) tightened up some aspects of the terms of service, for example the requirement for GPs to make themselves available on a regular basis throughout the working week. This formalised conditions of service in a way that removed ambiguity and exposed practices to challenge. Where the service received is felt to be unsatisfactory, the patient can pursue the matter in a formal complaint, initially to the practice. In more serious cases, most commonly claiming professional negligence, patients may become litigants. The creation of clearer responsibilities and standards of care is an important element in addressing imbalances between professional and client, although the drive of government initiatives has generally been the advancement of performance indicators benefiting practice populations. A somewhat impotent exception to this was the *Patient's Charter* (NHSME 1992b).

In tandem with its policies aimed at securing cost-effectiveness, the Conservative government in the 1980s and 90s attempted to graft consumerist measures onto the state-funded NHS and exhorted health authorities to consult more frequently with local communities (NHSME 1992a). *The New NHS* (DoH 1997) and the White Papers for Wales and Scotland indicated that the Labour government would similarly support consumerist approaches to enhance patient influence, including the use of consumer surveys on general practice as well as on hospital and community services' performance. Policy implementation may not, however, always match the aspirations or the rhetoric of policy-makers. Many factors impinge on successful policy implementation, from existing and perhaps immutable conditions to the reaction of the health service workers, Lipsky's (1980) street-level bureaucrats, and to the often unseen or uncalculated elements elsewhere in the system that conspire either to expedite, transform or diminish the impact of policy.

Consumerism, Markets and Contracts

The creation of CHCs in 1974 was the first major attempt to represent the views of the consumer in the NHS. Several policy initiatives in the 1980s signalled the government's intention to create a more consumer-responsive health service, an objective that has to be seen as the necessary adjunct of a more marketised provision and the mechanism by which providers are ultimately disciplined. The White Paper *Working for Patients* (DoH 1989a) indicated general practice's involvement in 'assisting patient choice' and the fact that it would itself 'need strengthening in four areas: *patient choice*; medical audit; prescribing costs; and management' (1989:54, emphasis added). The main focus of the White Paper was the hospital sector, but one measure that attracted a great deal of interest was the introduction of GP fundholding, an attenuated form of consumerism in which responsibility for referral decisions still remained with the GP.

Measures designed to make GPs more responsive to patients had already been proposed in an earlier White Paper, *Promoting Better Health* (DHSS 1987). The improvement in standards was to be achieved mainly by increased monitoring of performance in general practice by the FPCs – a bureaucratic arrangement. A market solution of sorts was evident in the proposals to require practices to provide information about themselves and to simplify the arrangements[1] for changing GPs, in Hirschman's (1970) terms, facilitating exit. The latter measure, coupled with the intention to increase the proportion of GPs' incomes delivered by capitation payments (related to the number and age of patients on a GP's practice list) was deemed to give some provider discipline. These arrangements were presumably predicated on several assumptions: that GPs would seek to sustain or maximise income despite costs (of time and effort) to them, and that increasing income from capitation, as opposed to other sources, would prove the most attractive strategy. Second, the proposals assumed that the desire to maintain or increase list size and the threat of patient exit would be converted into improved performance through a fear of losing patients. Finally, they assumed that providing patients with more information and an easier method of exit would make them more informed and active consumers. These hypotheses deserve closer scrutiny.

The relationship between payment type and GP behaviour is complex and somewhat underresearched (Krasnik 1990, Calnan and Hutten 1992). In the UK, this complexity is underscored by the fact that GPs are paid by both capitation and items-of-service fees. The 1990 GP contract reduced or removed some routine payments to GPs (for example a basic practice allowance and seniority payments) and replaced them with a system that offered proportionately greater rewards for those practices which increased their list size and could demonstrate activity in certain areas, such as health promotion and minor surgery, or reach specified targets in screening and immunisation. The assumption, supported by some within the profession (Morrell 1989), was that this would encourage larger lists. There is some evidence, albeit generated from a different health care system, indicating that doctors adjust their behaviour to achieve a target income (Rice 1983, Rosen 1989), and Mechanic (1975) has suggested that doctors paid on a capitation basis will work faster while those reimbursed on a 'fee-for-service' basis will work for longer periods, presumably stimulated by the thought of more patient contacts and a greater volume of fees. In their study of GPs in the UK and the Netherlands, Calnan and Hutten (1992) observed that any increase in list size resulting from the change in reimbursement might produce a deterioration in the quality of care because of the tendency to reduce consultation length as well as the time spent on such things as administration, planning and postgraduate education. Evidence from an earlier study by Calnan and Butler (1988) suggests a complicated relationship between list size and GP workload, which indicated their ability to exercise considerable discretion in organising work activities.

UK GPs may, however, choose not to compete to increase list size but instead to maximise income from 'items of service'. While there is a relationship between list size and income opportunities from such sources as minor surgery and health promotion, it could be assumed that GPs might prefer to sustain or enhance income by preferentially maximising non-capitation income from stable lists. Fee-based (non-capitation) income might represent a more controllable element within general practice, as opposed to the less predictable additional demand for consultations, such as home and out-of-hours visits, generated by larger lists. In addition, the generation of fee-based income from items such as cervical smears and immunisation and vaccination clinics can be delegated to other, less expensive staff. All things considered, the consumerist premise of the 1990 GP contract – that an increase in capitation payments would stimulate a more competitive spirit among GPs and ultimately improve services to patients – is unsubstantiated.

There has in fact been a gradual decline in average list size, something that the profession's leaders have encouraged. In the 1985–95 period, the average list size of unrestricted principals in England declined from 2,059 in 1985 to 1,885 in 1996 (DoH 1998c). In Scotland, Wales and Northern Ireland, the average list size has traditionally been smaller. Despite this, the demand for consultations between 1983 and 1993 rose slightly, GP principals undertaking on average an additional 436 consultations per annum by 1993. This may in part be the result of an increase in the proportion of patients over the age of 75 on GP lists (OHE 1995), but whatever the cause, the gradual increase in demand for consultations undoubtedly contributes to a prevailing view among GPs that their workload is increasing.

More specifically, evidence is accumulating of increasing pressure of work as a result of the GP contract, particularly in relation to administrative duties (Hannay *et al.* 1992, Chambers and Belcher 1993, Spurgeon *et al.* 1995), a perception that is echoed in the popular medical press. Evidence of the impact of the NHS internal market is, according to Pedersen and Leese (1997), less convincing. In their examination of studies on the effects of the shift of care to the community, they excluded research whose methodology could not differentiate between workload associated with the shift in the balance of care and that which would have existed in any case. With the exception of one study, which examined the discharge of long-stay mental patients into the community, they concluded that the knock-on effect was minimal. The internal market and now PCGs and LHGs have, however, created additional administrative responsibilities for GPs. Given these circumstances, it could be hypothesised that the average partnership might prefer to maintain or even slightly reduce its average list size and seek other ways of controlling work-loads, a logic that contradicts the consumerist tactics of the 'new' GP contract.

Other factors may conspire to reduce patient choice beyond a general wish to constrain list size growth. Conventions operate that serve to ease the pressure of work. Writing before the introduction of the reforms, Leavey *et al.* (1989) identified these as the drawing of practice boundaries, a reluctance to accept patients leaving another practice and the exclusion of some categories of undesirable patient. Overlaying this is the moderate control (inducement or prohibition) exerted over the distribution of GPs by the MPC according to whether an area is under- or overprovided with GPs. This has had the beneficial effect of ironing out grosser inequalities that existed between undersupplied and adequately supplied areas, although Bartlett (1996) reports that the variance of list sizes between regional health authorities increased between 1982 and 1993 (see Chapter 6 for a further discussion of equity in provision). Controls over recruitment to medical schools and a regulatory rather than market-generated distribution of GPs, however, has meant that no areas approach saturation and GPs therefore do not struggle to compete on the basis of insufficient patient number.

Even if GPs reject past practice and professional etiquette and aggressively compete to increase list size, there is little to suggest that this might be converted into improved patient care – a stated objective of the consumerist measures. There appears to be an inverse relationship between list size and the length of the consultation (Wilkin and Metcalfe 1984, Calnan and Butler 1988, Howie *et al.* 1989). The prevailing view among the academic leadership of the profession is that consultations of inadequate length achieve little (Tudor Hart 1995). Despite the length of consultation being in itself a crude measure, Howie *et al.* (1989) found that longer consultations tended to result in greater attention to psychosocial problems and a reduced prescribing of antibiotics, implying a more considered approach to diagnosis and treatment. The authors' research also noted that patient complaints tended to focus on insufficient time spent with the doctor and inadequate explanation of the diagnosis and treatment. More recently, Williams and Calnan (1991) also found that, against high general levels of expressed satisfaction with primary care, 24 per cent of the patients sampled were dissatisfied with the length of time spent in consultation, 26 per cent were dissatisfied with the level of information they received, and 38 per cent felt that they could not discuss their personal as opposed to medical problems with GPs. The study did not explore patients' conceptualisations of personal as opposed to medical problems, but, given the emphasis within the profession on an holistic approach and the consultation as a opportunity for patients to define their problems (May *et al.* 1996), it seems reasonable to assume that 'personal problems' might legitimately fall within the scope of the consultation. While longer consultations might not automatically deliver the goods for consumers of health care, they might at least increase the likelihood of a satisfactory consultation.

Patients' assessments of the performance of their doctor may not be that discerning. In Lloyd *et al.*'s (1991) study of Australian patients and primary care, the attributes of a 'good' doctor were related to affective characteristics, followed by the clinical competence of the doctor and her or his accessibility. Lloyd *et al.* concluded that the majority of patients in the study did not demonstrate consumerist attitudes or behaviour. Other studies consistently show general levels of satisfaction but dissatisfaction with specific areas (Cartwright and Anderson 1981, Fitzpatrick 1984, Williams and Calnan 1991). Displeasure is, however, rarely converted into action. The number changing practice for reasons other than a change of address tend to be small (personal communication, NHSE 1998; see also Billingshurst and Whitfield 1993, Thomas *et al.* 1995). In the Australian study, the reluctance to change doctor was particularly the case with elderly patients. Thus, the threat of exit that operates in commercial markets seems less applicable in general practice.

An effective consumer is someone who acts rationally on the basis of information about the costs and quality of health care and is able and motivated to exercise choice (Shackley and Ryan 1994). Some of the limitations to choice have already been discussed, but for those patients who are able to choose between practices, there are additional difficulties related to the quality of information. In a modest attempt to address this imbalance, an initiative to encourage practice charters was begun, as a part of the wider *Patient's Charter*, in November 1992 (NHSME 1992b). All charters were required to contain a statement of patients' rights, which varied from the rather obvious right to be registered with a GP to less familiar ones, such as the ability to choose whether or not to take part in medical research or medical student training. As well as collaborating with members of the wider primary health care team in the creation of local charters, practices were encouraged to incorporate the 'Users' Guide to Primary Health Care' (EL(92)88 Annex D). This duly reminded patients of their responsibilities (for example keeping appointments and requesting only essential night and home visits) as well as establishing a series of service commitments, the first of which stated that the patient 'will be treated as a partner in the care and attention (s/he) receives' (op. cit.). Finally, the NHSME guidelines indicated the need to establish standards in relation to access, contact and arrangements for dealing with suggestions and complaints.

Although no specific incentives have been approved nationally, the practice among many health authorities has been to offer financial support for the production of the mandatory practice leaflets where these have included information relevant to the local charter initiative. In numerical terms, progress with the initiative has been significant, 85 per cent of practices having developed or being in the process of developing charters by March 1997. However, the relative success of health authorities in persuading GPs to produce local charters has varied from 100 per cent (six health authorities) to 60 per cent or less (four health authorities), the lowest being 51 per cent (personal communication, DoH 1998). Furthermore, although individual health authorities may monitor the content, there does not appear to be a national evaluation of performance framed by the standards set in practice charters or the extent to which the sentiments expressed in 'Users' Guide to Primary Health Care' have been incorporated.

As indicated above, all practices have since 1990 had to provide information about such items as surgery times and the services available. While practice leaflets may produce information that allows some patients to discriminate more effectively between practices, for example on whether the practice includes a woman doctor, this may not always be the case. More problematic is placing information in the public domain that would inform potential patients about the quality of the service provided. What might be described as the technical competence of doctors – their ability to diagnose accurately and treat appropriately on a consistent basis – is difficult for laypersons to assess. This contributes to an asymmetry of information, which weakens consumer leverage in health care. Patients may be more likely to form an impression of quality in general practice based on a different set of criteria. In Billinghurst and Whifield's (1993) study, the avoidable practice characteristics that caused patients to change their doctor (for example long waiting times, a lack of continuity of care, rude receptionists and a lack of confidence in the doctor) might be considered as such. Patients in Williams and Calnan's (1991) study also most frequently reported waiting times in surgeries as a cause of dissatisfaction. These complaints are, with the exception of waiting times, difficult to assess objectively and might therefore prove difficult to incorporate in any institutionalised assessment of a practice's performance.

The focus on public information and formal processes might underestimate the information-gathering and assessment that takes place informally. Salisbury's (1989) study identified, among other things, that before selecting a GP, 51 per cent of the sample tried to find out about the practice from friends, relatives, workmates, neighbours or previous householders; a further 40 per cent, however, did not make any effort to seek out information before joining a practice. Salisbury concluded that patients showed little inclination to find out information from existing (formal) channels and that they exercised little active choice, although it is possible to interpret these results differently. Moreover, Salisbury's study preceded the creation of the internal market in health and the growing emphasis on consumerism.

More proactively, some general practices have undertaken informal patient satisfaction surveys, but it is difficult to ascertain how routine or widespread this practice is. Patient involvement in medical audit within general practice should aim at robust and constructive assessments of performance rather than satisfaction surveys. The content and process of audit within the NHS is, however, largely controlled by the medical profession and has therefore tended to focus on clinical performance rather than aspects of administration or communication. The DoH has endorsed user involvement in clinical audit, most recently in its consultative document *A First Class Service* (1998b), which covers England. Northern Ireland, Wales and Scotland will presumably devise their own systems.

Closer to general practice, Newton (1996) notes the Primary Health Care Clinical Audit (PHCCA) Working Group's recommendation that the views of service users be incorporated into clinical audit and, moreover, that the values of service users should be reflected in the criteria of measurement. This approach is also strongly endorsed by the Scottish Consumer Council (1997). Research focusing on general practice is difficult to locate, but two research studies (cited by Kelson and Redpath 1996) have reported a low level of lay membership on health authority Medical Audit Advisory Groups and Trust Clinical Audit Committees, the bodies largely responsible for promoting audit within the NHS. Membership is only the first stage. Capturing the agenda – at least a part of it – is an important element of true participation. The PHCCA Working Group could only recommend and cajole;

for the present, patients and consumer groups appear to have made little impact on the extent and focus of medical audit in general practice.

A further indication of consumerism, albeit reactive and frequently considered negative in form, is the trend in complaints made about the NHS and general practice. In recent years, the complaints process has been emphasised as the main mechanism of ensuring accountability to patients (Lupton *et al.* 1998), leading to a diminished role for the independent CHCs (Millar, cited in Lupton *et al.* 1998). Confidence in the data has been compromised by incomplete returns over a number of years up to 1996, making quantitative analysis problematic. Table 8.1 below is therefore difficult to interpret, but, overall, there appears to have been a slow increase in the number of complaints during this period.

The rhetoric on consumerism surrounding the creation of the internal market, the publication of the *Patient's Charter* (NHSME 1992b) and the awareness of standards have heightened the general public's expectations. It could be predicted that complaints about health care professionals would increase, not least because of a simplification in the complaints process. In May 1994, a government-appointed committee established to review the previously labyrinthine and highly defensive complaints procedure in the NHS published its proposals. The recommendations of *Being Heard* (DoH 1994) were accepted by the government (DoH 1995). These required all GP practices and NHS trusts to have, by April 1996, their own complaints procedures in place, with an emphasis on accessibility, swiftness, informality and fairness to all involved. Wherever possible, complaints were to be resolved at this stage by explanation and, if appropriate, by an apology and a review of practice processes. If the complainant remained dissatisfied with the practice's response, she or he would be entitled to request an independent review committee of the health authority. Decisions to grant independent reviews are taken by convenors who

Table 8.1 Number of resolved informal complaints and formal complaints to the Medical Service Committee for England and Wales, 1991/92–1995/96

Type of complaint	1991/92	1992/93	1993/94	1994/95	1995/96
Informal/resolved	2,188[1]	2,134[1]	2,776	2,468	1,930
Formal	1,537[1]	1,776[1]	1,944	1,901	1,938

Source: Department of Health, General Medical Census, Additional Data Collections 1994/95 and 1995/96.
Notes

1. Welsh data not available.

Table 8.2   Written complaints about Medical Services (Family Health Services) in England and Wales, 1996/97 and 1997/98

	Total written complaints	Cases requesting independent review	% of cases requesting independent review	Cases referred to I.R. panel	% of cases referred to I.R. panel
1996/97					
England	30,586[1]	776[1]	2.5[1]	184[1]	0.6[1]
Wales	1,456[2]	28[2]	1.9[2]	20[2]	1.4[2]
1997/98					
England	31,199[1]	1,086[1]	3.5[1]	286[1]	0.9[1]
Wales	1,463[2]	41[2]	2.8[2]	13[2]	0.9[2]

Notes

1. General Medical Census Additional Data Collections 1996/97 and 1997/98. Department of Health, *Handling Complaints; Monitoring the NHS Complaints Procedures 1996–97 and 1997–98*.
2. *Health Statistics: Wales 1998*.

are generally non-executive officers of the health authority. In addition, the health service commissioner's responsibilities were extended to include complaints against GPs, and the time limit within which a complaint could be registered was increased from 13 weeks to 12 months. The health service commissioner could also receive complaints from individuals dissatisfied with the original response. Table 8.2 gives the number of complaints, at the various stages of the process, for England and Wales.

In Scotland, complaints about medical primary care services[2] numbered 2,165 in 1996/97 and 2,042 in 1997/98. As in England and Wales, the system is based on the *Being Heard* document. Most complaints in Scotland were dealt with at the local level, only 4–5 per cent of cases progressing to the independent review stage. Two-thirds of these were concerned with clinical aspects of care, the remainder relating to communication difficulties (Scottish Office Department of Health 1998). The small number of complaints compared with those received in England and Wales no doubt reflects differences in population size, but even when this is taken into consideration, the number of complaints per person in Scotland is lower than that in England and Wales (personal communication, Scottish Executive 1999).

It is too soon to provide any firm indication of how well the new complaint system is working. Its lack of formality at the initial stage does appear to strengthen the hand of patients, and early impressions from the health service commissioner indicate that many complaints are dealt with satisfactorily at the local level, although, of those complainants dissatisfied with the outcome of this stage, few were granted the independent review they requested (Buckley 1997). A more recent study was critical of the system. In particular, it identified problems in primary care in that patients were daunted by the prospect of complaining to the practice directly and fearful of reprisals (Wallace and Mulcahy 1999). Familiarity with and a dependency on the subject of one's prospective complaint is a powerful discouragement to proceed. Supporting a climate in which complaints can be made freely but responsibly is a matter for the NHS as a whole and health authorities in particular.

The large number of written complaints received about medical services in England and Wales since 1996 undoubtedly reflects the improved collection of data in a more accessible system (written complaints made to practices in the first instance) rather than an exponential growth in the level of dissatisfaction. The upward trend in complaints over several years is, however, more indicative of a disjuncture between the rising expectations of the general population and what the service, including general practice, is able or willing to offer. Ultimately, for those patients who feel that they have a serious grievance and are not appeased by internal health service processes, there is a recourse to law. Both the Medical Defence Union (MDU) and the Medical Protection Society have experienced a rise in the number of complaints and claims. The MDU estimates a '15 per cent per annum (frequency and amount) increase' in claims of medical negligence (personal communication, MDU 1997). The increasing recourse to litigation may reflect a dissatisfaction with the normal complaints process or the development of a more aggressively consumerist and less indulgent culture among patients. To the degree that it is attributable to the former, a more responsive and open complaints process may head off litigation, with its damaging financial consequences for the NHS.

Patient Participation and General Practice

While consumerist strategies to improve access, choice, the amount and quality of information and the process of making a complaint have been evident in government policy in relation to general practice, the latter has been silent on the more volatile topic of patient participation. In its most robust form, patient participation requires an involvement with decision-making at each stage of the process, from the creation of an agenda to decisions about appropriate objectives and strategies. It owes more to democracy than consumerism, but was an element within the general movement for consumer rights and professional accountability in health care signalled by the creation of the Patients Association in 1963. The WHO initiative has more recently provided an additional impetus to patient and community participation in primary care. In the UK, this ethos has been partially evident within the Healthy Cities, Healthy Alliances and Health Action Zones initiatives.

Local Voices represents the Conservative government's exhortation to health authorities to become 'champions of the people' (NHSME 1992a:2). Its flamboyant language hints at the underlying process, that of consultation with and, if appropriate, the promotion of a community or group's view, rather than participation *per se*. Whatever outcomes for health authority consultation exercises were anticipated, *Local Voices* neglected to mention consultation by general practices. More radical elements in general practice had, however, already accepted the concept of patient participation groups, the first of which were established in the early 1970s. According to one source, growth was slow, and at the time there were estimated to be 131 practices with some form of patient representation (Mant, personal communication cited in Agass *et al.* 1991). The authors do not indicate whether this figure relates to the UK as a whole or any part, but, in comparison with the 25,257 partnerships[3] in England and Wales in 1990 (DoH 1998c), these figures demonstrate the relative paucity of the movement.

A difficulty encountered might be patchy health authority support for such developments, one exception being the Fife Health Board. Elsewhere in Scotland, limited development has occurred, this largely because 'a particular GP has supported the idea, or more generally, as a result of circumstances' (Scottish Consumer Council 1997:32). The concept of participation is variable, some practices harnessing patients' efforts in fund-raising or volunteering, others involving patients in planning services (see, for example, Heritage 1994). Neve and Taylor are similarly critical of the lack of success, declaring that 'existing methods... tend to be one off events, and are rarely central to planning' (1995:524). Even if GPs are willing to commit resources to establishing and running participation groups, there remains the difficulty of maintaining momentum (Scottish Consumer Council 1997). Additionally, Agass *et al.* point out that the limited development of the movement has been compounded by a high rate of disbandment. Although not offering solutions, Pietroni and Chase (1993) concluded from their experience of a patient participation group at a London health centre that it was important to define roles clearly, as expectations are likely to differ. They found patients to be disappointed that they had not been involved in real decision-making, while the staff expressed concerns about confidentiality, the professional–patient boundary and the small number of patients involved in what was deemed to be a representative process. This last finding is supported by Agass *et al.* who report that only 7 per cent of those practice patients responding had ever attended a patient group meeting. The colonisation of patient participation forums by the articulate, professional and semi-professional groups, and the relative lack of GP involvement, were factors deemed to have contributed to groups' failure elsewhere (Mann, cited in Agass *et al.* 1991).

Such difficulties are not readily overcome. At the very least, they would require GPs to commit more time and resources when a common perception of the profession is that the workload of GPs has risen inexorably (see, for example, Iliffe and Haug 1991, Chambers and Belcher 1993, Leese and Bosanquet 1996). In addition, it is probable that there is some resistance to the principle of patient participation groups, the rationale for which extends from the fear of such processes being taken over by 'frequent practice attenders... the unhappily married... and a task force of militant tendency' (*Lancet*, 1981:239), to the more sober but equally unyielding view of general practice as an independent concern that, accordingly, should be organised and run with the least possible interference from NHS managers or the public. More encouragingly, there are signs that the current emphasis on lay participation in service planning is being matched by a profession-led initiative encouraging partnership with patients (see Cleary 1999, Coulter 1999, Gafni 1999, Williamson 1999).

Professional and Policy Approaches – a Synergy?

It would be wrong to give the impression that a reluctance to involve patients in decisions about services offered by GPs and the primary health care team is necessarily symptomatic of a more widespread cynicism surrounding the patients' role or their rights. The profession itself has tried to import a less paternalistic and, in principle, more open quality to patient consultations that might at first sight seem compatible with consumerist policies in health care. However, the more adult and egalitarian approach that might characterise the consultation styles of some practitioners has little direct relationship with the culture of consumerism encouraged by the purchaser–provider split or the terms of the 1990 GP contract. Professional–client relationships in private markets are reinforced by contract and direct payments; within UK general practice, they are increasingly framed by resource constraints.

In competitive markets, the search for profits theoretically encourages the pursuit of efficiency without sacrificing quality; consumer perceptiveness and awareness is seen as a necessary condition of this. This chapter has already reviewed some of the evidence concerning consumer strength in the NHS, but a further difficulty is that service quality has had to be maintained within finite resources and against perceived increases in demand. Unpopular decisions inevitably have to be made, which are open to challenge by an increasingly sophisticated element within the patient population. Furthermore, the ability of the articulate, educated, health-seeking patient to secure a disproportionate share of resources may, ironically, be enhanced by a greater emphasis on effective treatment outcomes and their association with healthy behaviours.

An insistence on consumer awareness may have been visited on a NHS whose culture, notwithstanding the inroads that post-Griffiths managerialism has made, still tends to objectify patients, dealing with them in a routinised manner. Despite characteristically post-Fordist attempts to fragment the bureaucratic production of health care into atomised producers and providers, the NHS remains concerned with, if not the mass production of health care, certainly production for the masses. Policy objectives, which seek to improve efficiency, reduce waiting lists and extract value for money, have been measured in the hospitals and community services sector in completed consultant episodes or waiting periods for initial outpatients appointments. The pressure, therefore, has been to increase the rate at which patients are seen and treated rather than necessarily improving the experience. While general practice is a more idiosyncratic form of health care production and has not been subject to the same performance reviews as the hospital and community services sector, it has inevitably been enveloped by changes in service culture.

Nevertheless, the attempts by the Conservative governments in the 1980s and 90s to raise the awareness of consumerism in the NHS have had some effect on general practice. Patients are, in principle, able to change GP more easily and should be able to obtain information on the practice more readily. An increasing awareness of standards in the NHS as a whole may encourage less tolerance of poor service, as reflected by the increase in the number of complaints, although this may also be because of a simplified and more accessible complaints procedure.

For GPs, patient satisfaction is a more complex achievement than formerly and not limited solely to bedside manner and/or clinical outcome, although this remains an important element. As a consequence, the increased emphasis on providing consumer-sensitive services creates a particular tension in general practice, which is not only the first point of contact that most patients have with the NHS, but also the only point of contact for many patients for most of their lives. The point is not merely that rising patient expectations have made a particular impression on primary care services but that the more robust manifestations of consumerism find little support in this, the most autonomous and idiosyncratic part of the NHS. A less directive approach to therapeutic relationships does not extend to an incursion into the 'business' of general practice. The 'independent contractor' status, the long-term commitment of most GPs, and the private as opposed to state ownership of premises have encouraged a possessiveness of, perhaps even a defensiveness concerning, the practice of general practice. Alternatively, and more prosaically, it might be that GPs feel that the essence of their work is clinical practice and that they have little time to devote to consumerist and other initiatives.

The tensions apparent in attempts to graft a more consumerist culture on to semi-independent practices operating within a publicly funded system may well be exacerbated in the future. Having secured the chair and majority membership of PCG boards, GPs – primarily in England[4] – will be comprehensively involved in the allocation of resources to services and client groups. Since they nominate GP members to boards, all GPs will bear a corporate responsibility for the decisions made by the PCG and will presumably be held responsible by patients. There is evident concern among GPs about being scapegoated for taking difficult prioritisation decisions, the solution for some being the involvement of local communities in debates (Marks and Hunter 1998, North *et al.* 1999). For some GPs, the new arrangements will inevitably bring into sharp conflict the traditional role of the doctor as an advocate for the individual patient, and the new 'corporate' obligation towards local communities; however, developments in other areas of general practice, such as 'out-of-hours' collectives and more flexible employment arrangements may in any case weaken traditional values. Amidst this speculation one certainty persists: the many-faceted relationship between GPs and their patients will continue to evolve.

Notes

1. Patients were previously required to approach both their existing GP, who signed the requisite form, and the FPC before registering with another doctor.
2. The data cover practice-employed personnel as well as GPs.
3. Partnerships are used as a proxy for practices; DoH data are not collected for 'practices'.
4. In Scotland and Wales, the influence of GPs in service development and resource allocation is less certain. In Northern Ireland, proposals in *Fit for the Future* (DHSS 1998), albeit not yet enacted, will give Primary Care Cooperatives the budget for commissioning not only health, but also social services, in partnership with between two and five other Primary Care Cooperatives.

9

General Practice, Health and Social Care – Histories and Challenges

All three White Papers, for England, Scotland and Wales (DoH 1997, Scottish Office Department of Health 1997, Welsh Office 1998b), place great importance on relationships between the health service and other local agencies. In England, *The New NHS*, the government's blueprint for the health services, is at pains to emphasise the replacement of the internal market with a system of 'integrated care, based on partnership' (DoH 1997:Section 1.3). Its vision of integrated care extends beyond the vertical axis between primary and secondary health services, to incorporate social care, housing and education services in an ambitious drive to reduce health inequalities, but specifically mentioned is the 'crucial issue' (DoH 1997:13) of improved integration across health and social care.

Health authorities will clearly play an important role in working with agencies such as housing and education, especially in the early years of the 10-year programme of NHS reforms signalled by the White Paper. PCGs, however, will need to establish effective relationships with social services departments as well as secondary care providers. In addition, the Health Improvement Programmes will involve initiatives with other agencies at locality level, which, as the PCGs mature, will require effective networks. In Wales, LHGs already include voluntary sector organisations as well as health care professionals and representatives from departments of social services. Welsh health authorities may retain responsibility for strategic relationships, but LHGs could generate more pluralistic debates concerning priorities and service developments locally than might occur in PCGs. Scotland's PCTs will be expected to participate in the Local Care Partnership initiative designed to break down the boundaries between health and social care. As in Wales, Health Boards will, however, for the present, have the major responsibility for promoting interagency collaboration.

This is a taxing agenda for all stakeholders, particularly those in PCGs charged with planning health care. The history of health and social care planning is one of occasional welcome oases of good practice, and of processes hampered by resource protectiveness and professional defensiveness. Not all initiatives are top-down and small-scale developments, driven by the goodwill and cooperation of local practitioners, have often fared better. The planning and operation of services to provide seamless care in the community will necessitate conditions that overcome past obstacles and establish good working relationships between professionals at a number of levels. This chapter will discuss the extent to which GPs, as PCG members as well as providers of care, are prepared for these challenges. It will review the histories of community care planning and of interprofessional relationships between GPs and others involved in either the commissioning of care or the operation of agreed practice protocols, including those working in secondary care services. Of equal importance is an exploration of 'adjunct' relationships in local PCG processes, contractual relationships existing alongside those prescribed by membership of a PCG, and also of a changing dynamic: the preferencing of professional over market discourses.

The Record of Collaboration

GPs have, until recently, had little exposure to interagency planning, but the past experience of health and social services authorities is instructive. The attempt to distinguish health and social care services, following the National Health Service Act 1973, brought with it the risk of mismanaged care. In a potentially far-reaching decision, public health departments were, along with district nursing and health visitor services, transferred to health authority control. From the mid-1970s, the policy emphasis on deinstitutionalisation made it imperative that the new services collaborated effectively. In this era of top-down, rational planning (Barnard *et al.* 1980), joint planning teams were established, their plans fuelled by relatively modest amounts of joint finance. Much energy was spent on finessing organisational process, but joint planning achieved very little. *Care in Action* (DHSS 1981b) reflected government dissatisfaction with this state of affairs, reiterating the need for coordinated and accessible community care services.

The lack of success of community care was noted in a series of official reports as well as research studies (Social Services Committee 1985, Audit Commission 1986, Webb and Wistow 1986, NAO 1987). Ineffective collaboration at both planning and operational levels was identified as an important cause of failure. Contributing to this generalised diagnosis were a number of organisational and cultural difficulties. At the planning level, the lack of co-terminosity between district health authorities and local authorities, following the disappearance of area health authorities in 1982, hindered progress. Furthermore, the pressure on local authorities' spending, coupled with gloomy predictions in relation to future allocations from central government, created a climate of uncertainty. Budget procedures and planning cycles were different, as were systems for ensuring accountability (Audit Commission 1986). There were difficulties associated with the process of hospital closure for long-stay patients with mental ill-health and with learning difficulties in that these patients often needed to be relocated into the community often before resources could be released (Social Services Committee 1985, Audit Commission 1986). The Audit Commission also observed that much of the attention of health authorities was focused on acute provision whereas social services authorities had to respond to the increasing legislation in child care. These items formed part of a constellation of difficulties that hindered progress, but the crucial issue, and one that remains unresolved today, was the need to agree the responsibility for and coordination of the various elements of continuing care for those with long-term illness.

The effective coordination of community care at the operational level is equally important. There are reports of successful co-working between health and social care agencies, including general practices (Audit Commission 1986, McKinstry 1987, Hudson *et al.* 1998), but the difficulties stemming from the different professional cultures evident at the interagency level were also potent in professional relationships between practitioners. According to Morris (1993:635), there was a history of poor relations between GPs and social workers:

> The two professions tend to be suspicious of each other, have little understanding of each other's roles, and have very different cultures. Social workers operate in teams, take measured approaches to problems and rarely take decisions on their own. GPs work mainly as individuals supported by primary care teams.

Huntington (cited in Dalley 1991) drew attention to the distinctive professional ideologies of social work and general practice. The goal of normalisation and successful social functioning of individuals espoused by social workers contrasted with the curative, systemic pathology-centred approach of the medical profession. Dalley's study of health and social care workers found that, in relation to several issues, GPs 'were located at one end of an ideological continuum with field level social workers at the other' (1991:169). They differed in their views about such fundamental issues as the worth of institutional care and the role of families in community care. Furthermore, professional groups on either side of the organisational divide between the NHS and social services had internalised views that celebrated the value of their own profession's contribution and tended to belittle that of others. Social workers were accused by GPs and hospital clinicians of having a lethargic and bureaucratic approach to urgent problems, a criticism echoed in recent research (Khan and Lupton 1999). Similarly, Higgins *et al.* (1995) reported that health care workers regarded social services staff as undisciplined and commented on the lack of training of many, while social services staff felt that health workers operated within a medical model of care and that their involvement with clients was less open-ended. Their social focus also differed. Twigg and Atkin (1995) found that social workers focused on the family as a unit whereas GPs tended to view the patient as an individual.

Despite these differences, there is evidence of understanding: GPs in one study expressed sympathy for the pressures that social workers faced (Khan and Lupton 1999), and, despite the differences she found, Dalley noted that those working in the field felt more allegiance to other professionals sharing the same pressures than they did to managers in their respective agencies. She concluded that it was difficult to predict how health and social care workers might respond to the community care agenda but that an emphatic joint commissioning approach enabled by the purchaser–provider divide might overcome 'tribal ties'.

There have been a number of views on the role that GPs might perform in community care, ranging from coordinators to more marginal participants and, more recently, potential joint commissioners of care. In debates preceding the 1974 reorganisation of the NHS, the view of the Gillie Report (MOH 1963) was that the GP should be seen as coordinator of health and welfare services in the community. This had been challenged by Titmuss, among others, who argued that GPs showed little inclination in this direction (Means and Smith 1994). It was perhaps fortunate that the idea of making GPs responsible for the coordination of welfare services for individuals as well as for their clinical practice was abandoned. Organisationally, GPs still operated at the periphery of the NHS and valued their independence (see Chapter 2). Furthermore, the new responsibilities generated by the community care initiative from the mid-1970s onwards far outstripped the capacity of GPs and their embryonic practice administrations. There was, in any case, challenge enough in establishing new primary health care teams.

Some percipient MOHs were the first to promote the attachment of nursing staff to practices in the late 1950s (Hasler 1992), an idea given official support by the Ministry of Health in 1963. The 1974 reorganisation opted for administrative tidiness and, having dislocated health visiting and district nurses from local authority administration, gave a further boost to the trend of practice attachment. There were disadvantages to the new arrangements. Although, on the one hand, reorganisation placed together key workers responsible for providing health care in the community, it also created a system that segregated the two major agencies responsible for community care.

The idea of primary health care teams grew from the not unreasonable assumption that the simple process of locating nurses, health visitors, midwives and, on occasions, social workers in general practices would improve the care of patients. Evidence suggests that the mere co-location of professionals improves the mutual understanding of their roles and increases the number of referrals (Thomas and Corney 1993). In addition, the Family Doctors' Charter encouraged the building of larger premises and made the employment of practice staff, including practice nurses, a viable option. Thus, primary health care teams became agglomerations of attached health authority staff and GP practice employees, GPs often assuming a leadership role. These arrangements were often counterproductive, and the Harding Report appealed for more collaboration and a clarification of roles in primary care (DHSS 1981a). Despite this, there is considerable evidence to suggest that the aspiration of more effective team functioning has not been realised (Bond *et al.* 1985, DHSS 1986a, Wiles and Robison 1994, West and Field 1995).

The Cumberlege Report's review of community nursing reflected the frustration of many nurses with the ineffectiveness of primary health care teams. It proposed the parallel organisation of nurses in neighbourhood teams covering 'patches', which would facilitate community profiling and proactive, collaborative working with local authorities, a concept that foreshadows the ideal of PCG/PCT locality-based planning. Less apocalyptically, Cumberlege made recommendations for the enhancement of teamworking, including written agreements of objectives and work to develop a better understanding of team members' roles. Those doctors who chose not to participate in such arrangements would 'receive only those nursing services which the neighbourhood nursing managers themselves decided to provide' (DHSS 1986a:36). As such, Cumberlege offered a challenge to the dominant conceptualisation of primary health care teams and, indeed, primary health care as framed by the prevailing model of general practice. There was, predictably, much GP opposition to the Cumberlege Report, and the idea of patchworking was quietly shelved.

Despite these and others' exhortations, the operationalisation of primary health care teams remains problematic. West and Poulton (1997) found that primary health care teams performed less favourably than multidisciplinary teams in other organisational settings on four measures: clarity of objectives, participation, task orientation and support for innovation. Since PCGs are likely to demand similar strengths, one wonders how GPs and other board members, including community nurses, will fare.

GPs and Community Care

Whereas many primary health care teams may leave much to be desired in terms of exemplary performance, it is probably reasonable to assume that, in most practices, systems are in place which ensure that the internal referral of patients between practice staff, community nurses and GPs, as well as communication about progress, takes place on a routine basis. The same cannot be so confidently predicted of communication with other services. The cultural and administrative divide between, and often the geographical separation of, primary health care teams and social workers has created additional problems for community care. These and other difficulties emerge in research generated from two key areas of professional practice: mental health care and child protection.

Corney (1995) points out that 98 per cent of those defined as mentally ill are registered with a GP. The extent of psychiatric morbidity in the population, the closure of long-stay psychiatric hospital beds since the late 1970s and the intractable nature of some mental illnesses have made mental health care a significant element in GPs' workloads. Sheppard's (1992) examination of contacts between GPs, social workers and community psychiatric nurses (CPNs) found that there were substantially more CPN–GP contact episodes than social worker–GP episodes. In both situations, the GP was unlikely to initiate contact. More positively, a survey by Thomas and Corney (1992), of staff attached to or employed by general practice and dedicated to the care or support of those with mental illness, confirmed that this is more commonplace than before, 50 per cent of practices indicating a link with a CPN and a further 21 per cent with a social worker. A smaller proportion had regular contacts with counsellors and clinical psychologists.

These findings reflect not only the greater number of mental health workers operating in the community as a result of the closure of long-stay hospitals, but possibly also the preferences of GP fundholders expressed in contracts with community health care trusts. The Audit Commission observed that fundholders were more likely to offer a range of services of all kinds, but, interestingly, social workers were 'more commonly found at non-fundholders' premises' (1986:34). Despite these hopeful trends, Corney (1995) suggests that the assumption that attachment is synonymous with teamwork is a false one; overall the record of collaboration between GPs and other agencies, such as social services, is poor.

In child protection work, too, collaboration between health and social services personnel has given cause for concern, as evidenced in a series of inquiries into the deaths of children following abuse (see, for example, Committee of Inquiry 1974, Panel of Inquiry 1989). Although GPs have not been regarded as core professionals in child protection (Birchall 1992), these being social workers, the police and paediatricians, they have a seminal role in the identification of child abuse. The work undertaken by Birchall and Hallett (cited in Birchall 1995) uncovered dissatisfaction over the absence of GPs from child protection conferences, while for their part, GPs complained about the lack of notice.

Further research on interprofessional collaboration in child protection identified similar frustrations, together with the view that social services were slow to respond to expressions of concern about particular cases (Lupton and Khan 1999). The same authors recorded that the most cited option that GPs expressed for improving relations was social worker attachment to the primary health care team. There was a dissonance between the expectations of other front-line professionals involved in child protection, who felt that GPs had an important role to play in all stages of the process, and the views of most GPs, who considered that their contribution related primarily to the identification of children at risk. Furthermore, many GPs identified health visitors as the key health professional involved in continuing child care procedures. Birchall (1995) also points to the pivotal role of the health visitor as an intermediary between various elements in child protection networks. In summarising her research with Hallett, Birchall concludes that these difficulties are not likely to be readily resolved. It may well be that health visitors are better equipped to manage the primary health services' contribution to child protection cases, and, as a consequence, the GP's involvement in the process beyond the stage of identification should be reconsidered. More germane to this discussion is Birchall's observation that the study indicated a distance between GPs and social workers in child protection.

Accounts of the history of child protection and, to a lesser extent, contact patterns in mental health care provide evidence of a less than satisfactory collaboration in care arrangements. There are, however, GPs who seem committed to developing ambitious community health services for specific client groups. One such project plan, sketched in a *British Medical Journal* article, proposed integrated health care for people with learning difficulties living in group homes (Kendrick and Hilton 1997). The concept did not appear to embrace social care arrangements, or if it did, neither social workers nor client advocates were included in a team involving a wide range of health care professionals. This multidisciplinary myopia will not suffice given the operational complexities of community care and the need to ensure that provision is not medicalised. However, neither should GP interest be spurned. Although the profession's debates over core services indicate a growing desire to exercise discretion over which categories of clients they treat, in the presence of what many GPs judge to be a relentless increase in the pressure of work, GPs are clearly actively involved in providing medical services for a growing number of vulnerable client groups. They will in future also be inevitably drawn into the planning of community care within PCG boundaries.

Deinstitutionalisation and Efficiency

It is apparent that GPs have become increasingly dissatisfied with the impact of community care policies and, more recently, the NHS and Community Care Act 1990 on their workload. From the early 1980s, social security board and lodging arrangements encouraged the reinstitutionalisation of patients discharged into the community to residential units and nursing homes, and enabled the closure of long-stay wards. Between 1976 and 1994, the number of non-psychiatric NHS beds for elderly people decreased from 55,600 to 37,500 (Glendinning and Lloyd 1998). GPs inherited responsibility for their care, which, *ipso facto*, meant that they were treating a greater proportion of patients with a higher level of dependency than previously. In addition, the 1990 GP contract required GPs to make annual assessments of patients over the age of 75.

Although advances in technology made shorter periods of hospitalisation feasible and increased the range and number of therapies deliverable by GPs, it was the impetus of internal markets, coupled with the need to demonstrate efficiency gains, that encouraged a permeability of the boundary between hospital and primary care. Additionally, the NHS and Community Care Act ended the financial incentive to locate vulnerable clients in residential or nursing homes, reinforcing the need for more intensive domiciliary-based packages of health and social care.

The perception of GPs was not simply that their workload had considerably increased (Leedham and Wistow 1992, BMA 1995a) but that they were being required to render services outside those which they were contractually obliged to provide. In particular, the General Medical Services Committee (GMSC) identified as non-core services the 'Medical care of highly dependent patients living in the community, often in nursing homes or residential homes', a category that included 'small residential homes where independent and usually mobile patients attend a variety of local practices for ordinary general medical care' (GMSC 1996:5). The guidelines observed that, although in the latter case GPs might consider that the care of these patients (that is, those with learning difficulties or mental health problems) fell within core GP work, it might in some circumstances be considered outside the terms of service. The GMSC was also critical of the expectation that GPs would care for highly dependent patients, of whom the elderly would form the greatest proportion.

This position, if actively promoted, has obvious consequences for the effective operation of services. The need for improved interagency working as a result of the NHS and Community Care Act's reinforcement of community care, particularly domiciliary-based care, is self-evident. The DoH has long been concerned that 'the caring services work effectively together, each recognising and respecting each others' contributions and responsibilities' (1989a:13). Research evidence is mixed. As lead agencies, social services departments were responsible for arranging flexible packages of care that would support those with the highest levels of dependency in their own homes or, failing that, within institutions in the community. The response from members of a series of focus groups, which included GPs, enabled Henwood (1995) to report improved working relationships between health and social services agencies. Front-line staff had adopted informal and often unsanctioned working practices in order to resolve issues. Strains were, however, evident over continuing care responsibilities, especially where clients demonstrated complex needs. This perhaps reflects not only the increasing resistance of GPs to workload shifts, but also agencies' desires to protect hard-pressed budgets. The 'winter pressure' monies injected into the NHS by the Labour government may subsequently have relieved some of the difficulties, but participants' views also reflected concerns over a general absence of integrated planning by health and social services agencies at local and national levels. In general, Henwood observed that there appeared to be intensifying strains between health and social care.

The role of primary health care services in community care is threefold: to bring cases to the attention of care managers, to cooperate in the assessment of cases and to collaborate in the care arrangements. Early evidence suggests that GPs felt insufficiently informed about the changing community care arrangements. Take Care Associates (cited by Leedham and Wistow 1992), and a later BMA survey (1995a) indicated that a disappointingly small proportion (58.4 per cent) of respondents confirmed that they had been made formally aware of local procedures of assessments – fewer still (45.6 per cent) had been made aware of procedures covering discharge. Given the centrality of the GP's role in identification and early assessment, these were worrying disclosures. Leedham and Wistow point out that most surveys of the elderly have uncovered a hidden 'iceberg' of medical and social need. It was anticipated that the annual assessments of the elderly population on a GP's list, as required by the 1990 contract, would improve the identification of those at risk in a methodical manner, but a study based in Rotherham found that GPs referred only 8.5 per cent of their assessed cases whereas nurses referred 25 per cent (Nocon 1993). Such inconsistencies in approach might suggest a need for a greater clarification of the threshold for referrals and hence a greater use of referral protocols, although the Rotherham findings may also have reflected uncertainties concerning the assessment procedure early in the reforms.

According to Leedham and Wistow (1992), there was broad agreement between the FHSAs, social services departments and GPs that the latter should not take the lead role in assessment. GPs expressed a reluctance to do so because of other work pressures, the lack of remuneration for the task and

GPs' lack of understanding of community care. Other reasons cited by the authors, presumably generated by social services or FHSA personnel, were the GPs' inability generally to comprehend the big picture and the embeddedness of the GP assessment in medical models of practice, a view that echoes Huntingdon's findings. A later survey of social services departments (Hudson *et al.* 1998) identified concerns that the disposition of GPs was unsympathetic to effective joint working. Respondents commented on GPs' intransigence, occasionally their interest in payment, which was seen as antithetical to the notion of joint working, and more generally the difficulty in engaging a contribution from GPs. The authors concluded that: 'if there is one weak professional link in the collaborative chain, it is that of GPs' (1998:15). Given the important role that GPs will have in PCGs, these studies do not bode well for the future of shared commissioning.

Joint Commissioning and GPs

The NHS and Community Care Act did not merely intensify the changing balance of care from long-stay and acute institutions to care in the community, in turn encouraging changes in the nature of clinical general practice, but also ushered in the new role of the GP purchaser. This was initially synonymous with that of fundholder, which, in the early phase of internal markets, focused on a narrow menu of acute and community health services. Health authorities had a health service monopoly of the joint commissioning role, a product of their historical involvement in joint planning, experience gained from the production of parallel community care plans with local authorities and the relative immaturity of fundholding, which limited the latter's functional capabilities and purchasing power. Health authorities gradually involved GPs in strategic purchasing arrangements, although, according to a BMA (1997:8) survey, the level of participation suggests they had an 'advisory' rather than an 'active' role. The same survey reported that 90 per cent of the health authorities responding had joint commissioning arrangements and, of these, 38 per cent reported the involvement of GPs. No information was provided on the nature of GP involvement, but a single, in-depth case study elsewhere found limited consultation over draft joint purchasing strategies and a general reluctance of GPs to become more involved in joint strategy planning (North 1997b).

Strategic joint commissioning aside, there was the potential to influence care in the community through contracts made with acute and community health care providers. There is, however, little evidence to suggest that this was a principal concern of GP purchasers, a situation that perhaps gave greater urgency to the need for social services departments to apprise GPs of the probable impact of their decisions. Eaton (1997) reported the widespread concerns of senior social services managers, which included difficulties of negotiation with both health authority and locality tiers, the absence of any formal arrangements for involving GPs in joint commissioning in many areas and, similarly, the absence of social services representatives on locality commissioning groups. Differences in values and professional culture were once again cited as reasons for liaison problems, social services managers expressing concern about the possibility that GPs might in time dominate social care commissioning.

In the light of some proposals in the consultation document *Partnership in Action* (DoH 1998a), this may not be that eccentric a notion. Social services managers' anxieties should be viewed in the context of the past record of interagency collaboration, noted earlier in this chapter, together with evidence suggesting that tensions remain over such issues as 'bed-blocking' and care packages for elderly people (Healy 1997). Others have indicated that GPs' level of understanding and expertise in commissioning, as opposed to the much simpler function of fundholding, is limited (McCulloch and Ashburner 1997) and that GPs appear to lack a detailed knowledge about community services (Gordon and Hadley 1996). Notwithstanding these apparent limitations, GPs have been inexorably drawn into debates about planning issues.

The need to incorporate non-fundholders as well as fundholders in joint commissioning[1] has been self-evident, compelled by the division of responsibilities in continuing care following discharge from hospital and by the centrality of all GPs in the management of vulnerable clients. The growth of locality commissioning and multifunds provided an additional opportunity for joint commissioning, although, as Poxton (1994) suggests, these initiatives demanded much careful work to develop relationships, establish priorities and identify the best way in which to proceed. Poxton hints here at the potentially large agenda facing locality commissioning projects, not all of which were endowed with funds and therefore the wherewithal to influence service change. Despite such difficulties, there are examples of joint commissioning initiatives and also of the involvement of community nurses in a small number of locality commissioning initiatives (Dixon *et al.* 1997).

The TPPs that got under way in April 1995 offered exciting new opportunities for joint commissioning to develop both integrated purchasing and an integrated provision of community services. Research undertaken as part of a national evaluation programme of TPPs found that 19 out of 53 TPPs were involved in developing continuing and community care services. A more detailed study of five of the projects indicated that joint activities were focused on operational matters and tended to respond to problems that TPPs identified at the level of individual patient care. None involved strategic needs assessment (Myles *et al.* 1998). Integrated purchasing took place in only one of the five case studies in which the TPP funded contingency social care arrangements during peak holiday times, but there was no joint or indicative budget for the project. The authors noted, however, that the prospect for integrated purchasing was improved in that four out of the five had begun work to eventually agree joint budgets for health and social care packages at practice level. Similarly, there was work towards integrated provision, intended to improve the alignment and operational success of health and social care teams in the community. Although these observations suggest a welcome collaboration over community care, the authors pointed out that there was no evidence of innovation; instead, the changes that the TPPs had made were extensions of past initiatives.

The fact that continuation rather than innovation characterised the ventures may be more a product of the TPPs' relative immaturity. Given more time, the cementing of relationships and greater self-assuredness, TPPs might have been more radical. Perhaps a more worrying factor, since TPPs were in many ways the progenitors of PCGs, is that over half of the 53 TPPs did not consider themselves to be actively engaged in the development of community care services. This is a level of insularity that PCGs cannot afford and underlines the evolutionary leap that they will have to make before they can fulfil expectations of their role in planning seamless community care services.

All Together Now? PCGs, GPs and Collaborative Relationships

The Labour government clearly set out with the intention of creating more pluralistic forums for decision-making at locality level. The White Paper *The New NHS* (DoH 1997) declared that local doctors and nurses 'would be in the driving seat in shaping services' (Section 2.4) and observed the need to forge stronger links with local authorities. PCGs were to have a governing body that included 'community nursing and social services as well as GPs' (Section 5.15). Community nurses, hitherto marginalised in commissioning, responded favourably (Hancock 1998). Although there was no guarantee of professional egalitarianism, stage 1 and 2 PCGs were originally to have a non-medical majority membership. In the weeks following the publication of the White Paper, the GMSC of the BMA lobbied hard for GP control of the PCGs and succeeded in extracting guarantees of GP chairs and majority membership of PCG boards from Alan Milburn, Minister for Health, much to the consternation of the nursing leadership (Kenny 1998).

In Scotland, Health Boards have control of the budget for health care, but the government hopes that GPs, via local cooperatives, will play a central role in directing and managing the SPCTs, on which is placed a requirement to work closely with providers of social work services and housing. There has been little Scottish Office prescription of the structure, function and role of the local cooperatives (Hopton and Heaney 1999), or of how they articulate with SPCTs and other agencies. The expectation seems to be that locally inspired initiatives will fill the policy void. The contrast with the more detailed activities south of the border, where GPs had all to play for in gaining political control, could not be more stark.

In England and Wales, the numerical superiority of GPs on PCGs (LHGs in Wales), their professional status and local influence means that they will dominate local decision-making processes, as they have done within primary health care teams. There is a danger that overassertiveness will destroy critical relationships with community nursing and social work. Moreover, a study undertaken by Marks and Hunter (1998) revealed concerns that the absence of teamwork in many practices provided a weak basis for effective collaboration in PCG work. Community nursing has particular difficulties in that its representatives are likely to be either employees of GPs (practice nurses) or employed by a community health trust that must negotiate local service agreements with PCGs. These dynamics may intrude on working relationships within PCGs, particularly where there are differences of opinion over, for example, professional role development or the need for change in community nursing services.

Social services representatives on PCGs may enjoy a less complicated relationship, but they may well have difficulty in establishing a common agenda. Research by Myles *et al.* (1998) suggests that the focus of joint commissioning within TPPs was problem-inspired and tended to be incremental rather than strategic. A focus on tangible objectives may, however, be a better initial strategy for those GPs whose knowledge of the broader community care agenda is limited – as was indicated in the study. More problematic for PCGs than confined commissioning horizons is the financing of integrated social and health care projects. Without clearly defined criteria of access, inappropriate cost shunts between health and social services may result, damaging future ventures (North 1998).

The emphasis in *The New NHS* (DoH 1997) on collaboration rather than competition may, however, help to dissipate some of the possible tensions in PCGs. A study of GP views on the White Paper, undertaken in the first few weeks following its publication, found GPs promoting the idea of professional collegiality in external and internal PCG relationships. They welcomed cooperation in place of what they perceived as divisions previously imposed by the market. This perspective also embraced other professionals, including community nurses and social workers (North *et al.* 1999). In addition, Myles *et al.*'s (1998) study of TPPs suggests that the relationships between GPs and social services departments were improving in four out the five case study sites. Thus, the record of past relationships may be instrumental in predicting future difficulties but should perhaps not be overemphasised.

The precise role of social services representatives on PCGs is, at the time of writing, unclear. Presumably, they are to act in an advisory capacity in commissioning decisions and should also ensure that arrangements for separately funded elements of community care services are underpinned by effective coordination between the NHS and other stakeholders in community care. The discussion document *Partnership in Action* (DoH 1998a), produced in September 1998, was conspicuously reticent on joint working between health and social services in stage 2 and 3 PCGs (stage 1 PCGs being considered to be advisory bodies to health authorities). PCTs are seen as providing 'unique opportunities for community health services, primary care and social services to co-ordinate the care they provide' (Section 3.10) and are as such viewed as potentially the most important area for improvement. The document proposes more flexible budgetary arrangements between local authorities and health authority and/or PCT (stage 4) level so that resources can be pooled to commission and provide services. It also identifies social services authorities, health authorities or PCTs as possible lead commissioners taking responsibility for commissioning both health and social care. How social services authorities or health authorities integrate such unified commissioning arrangements with shared commissioning initiatives at the level of stage 2 and 3 PCGs is not explained. The absence of responsibility for stage 2 and 3 PCGs in the consultation document may reflect government concerns that they will not have attained a sufficient level of sophistication and expertise in joint commissioning relationships, or that they will be heavily committed to the remainder of their commissioning agenda, or both. Whatever the rationale, it will be important for health authorities or social services authorities to incorporate PCG initiatives in their plans. Similarly, PCTs will need to liaise closely with other stakeholders to ensure that parallel commissioning initiatives are coordinated.

PCGs will be central to integrated commissioning initiatives in the future, whether acting on their own volition or under the steerage of health authorities. GPs, as pivotal members of these influential organisations, will play a critical role in the success or failure of such ventures, the outcomes of which will also influence their role as service providers. However, they inherit responsibility for an area of policy more conspicuous for failure of collaboration than success. As a professional group, they also bring a history characterised in the main by independence rather than inter-reliance and effective teamwork, and by a degree of ignorance about community care policies at both national (Myles *et al.* 1998) and local level (Leedham and Wistow 1992).

PCGs will undoubtedly continue to try and 'fix what is broke' at the operational level, and this will hopefully cement relationships that form the basis of more adventurous interagency initiatives in the future, although *Partnership in Action* indicates the need for health authorities and local authorities to continue to lead commissioning in this area in the near and mid-future. With an imaginative use of the pooled budgets described in the discussion document to develop services at PCG level, a more strategic vision among PCG boards could, however, be encouraged. GPs will need help to develop expertise in this, perhaps the most difficult of tasks.

Notes

1. Joint commissioning can be defined as the coordination of health and social care planning through the sharing of information and/or expertise and the agreement of service priorities. It may, in addition, involve the shared (although not pooled) funding of jointly 'owned' programmes.

10

Conclusion – Comparisons and Futures

The preceding chapters have provided an analysis of the current policy issues facing general practice in the UK. The assessment began with a consideration of the historical context from which contemporary general practice has evolved. Attention then focused on the two issues that have framed general practice today and provided the contemporary context for its present significance within UK health care policy as a whole. These were the development of the 1990 GP contract and the emergence of the GP role in health care commissioning. Subsequent chapters then explored the implementation and implications of these developments with regard to the spatial provision of general practice to under-doctored and deprived areas, general practice in urban and rural areas, the accountability of GPs, and the relationship between GPs and their patients as well as between GPs and other agencies, most notably those involved in social care.

The purpose of this concluding chapter is to stand back from the analysis of day-to-day developments in general practice and take a broader view of ways in which general practice in the UK might evolve in the future. Two distinct perspectives are taken. First, an assessment is offered of the extent to which the experience of general practice in other countries can provide an indication of possible developments in the future UK context. For reasons that will be outlined below, three countries have been selected for attention: New Zealand, the USA and the Netherlands. The second part of the chapter considers the future from the internal UK position. There is a brief reprise of the probable implications of the further extension of the current system of a 'primary care-led NHS'. Attention then shifts to an analysis of alternative ways of organising and financing primary care delivery. This discussion includes reference to private and insurance-based general practice.

A Comparative Perspective

A key purpose of comparative analysis is the uncovering of points of similarity and dissimilarity between, in this case, systems of general medical practice. From this emerges the objective of identifying lessons that may be transferred between settings. Unreasoned and random comparisons are seldom helpful, however, providing little beyond a generalised finding that things are done differently in different places. For this reason, effective comparative analyses usually begin from positions of similarity between systems or societies. This is the strategy behind the section of the case studies presented here. There are important points of similarity between the chosen case studies and the UK situation.

New Zealand

New Zealand provides the first case study. The points of comparison here are twofold. First, the overall New Zealand health care system bears a considerable resemblance to that of the UK. A publicly-funded NHS has been the subject of New Right reforms in the early 1990s. Indeed, as Cumming and Salmond (1998) report, New Zealand drew explicit lessons from the UK experience. Second, the post-reform New Zealand policy experience has provided an important basis for other countries seeking to develop a 'post-welfare state' (Kelsey 1995). In particular, the UK New Labour project has drawn on the New Zealand approach. It might thus be hypothesised that what has happened and is happening in New Zealand provides an indication of the way in which things may evolve in the UK.

In New Zealand, GPs act as gatekeepers to secondary care in much the same way as their UK counterparts do. Unlike the situation in the UK, New Zealand patients are, however, allowed to move readily between GPs and do not have to stay with the same GP for successive consultations: they can 'doctor-shop' (Barnett and Kearns 1996). A more important contrast, however, is that New Zealand GPs are essentially private providers of general medical services. Patient use of general practice in the New Zealand health service is funded principally by direct payments by patients and fee-for-service subsidies from the public exchequer (Fougère 1993). Patients cover the gap between the government subsidy and the full primary care fee through private health insurance (Cumming and Salmond 1998). From a patient perspective, it is therefore a quasi-private service and is fiscally distinct from the tax-funded hospital system.

The result of these separate financial regimes was, prior to the reforms, a lack of integration between the sectors. In the context of general practice, the financial regime, especially the subsidy element, was such that there was little control over GP activity. Government expenditure on general practice increased through the 1980s (Malcolm 1993). The then Labour government increasingly embraced New Right perspectives in its attempt to halt this cost escalation and end the lack of integration between primary and secondary care. Familiar measures were enacted, including the introduction of prescription charges, voluntary contract schemes whereby GPs received enhanced state subsidies provided they agreed to limit their fees, and the employment of salaried GPs to ensure 24-hour coverage in areas of high health care need but little financial attraction to GPs.

The 1990 National government continued this process, and a purchaser–provider split emerged bearing close similarity to that of the UK model of the internal market as it was consolidated in 1995/96. Four regional health authorities were initially created to purchase care from private and public health care providers. The funding for the regional health authorities took the form of an integrated budget for both primary and secondary care. On the provision side, GPs were expected to enter into contracts with a regional health authority (Barnett and Barnett 1997). The balance between fees-for-service and government subsidy shifted in favour of the former. Cumming and Salmond (1998) record how the four regional health authorities had, by the mid-1990s, metamorphosed into a single Health Funding Agency and made significant progress in setting up contracts with GPs. By mid-1996, half of all GPs had devolved budgets for support services, and one-fifth had moved to capitation contracts.

The contractual relationships between GPs and purchaser authorities were predicated upon a purchaser goal of curbing expenditure. Accountability was also, in a way strongly reminiscent of the 1990 UK GP contract, to be enhanced by means of performance measurement and performance standards. Further goals included the promotion of service integration between primary and secondary care through a limited form of GP budget-holding (a parallel with UK GP fundholding) and limitations on practice provision in over-doctored areas (a analogy with the UK MPA policy). The practical implications of this arrangement for GPs had two aspects. On the one hand, there was a distinct loss of autonomy. Choices of where to practise were reduced, and incomes became tied to performance in a way that had never been the case in the previous dispensation. On the other hand, the potential to become a budget-holder offered the possibility of innovative service developments, and the constitution of GPs as a provider entity contrasted with the regional health authority purchasers gave an important sense of identity and provided a basis for cooperation and collaboration.

This latter impact has been particularly marked. It underpinned the formation of independent practice associations (Malcolm and Powell 1996). These are groupings of GPs coming together to pool their interests with regard to economies of scale, risk-sharing and contract negotiations with the purchaser authority. In effect, these represent the creation of a cooperative response on the part of the GPs to the pressures stemming from the introduction of the internal market. They offer the possibility of mutual protection, yet they also have wider implications. Although there might be arguments to the contrary, general practice in a private sector environment seldom fosters strong mutual allegiances between patient and GP. The emergence of independent practice associations has helped the development of greater community linkages. While patients may doctor-shop between individual GPs, they usually restrict their 'shopping' to within the independent practice association. In this way, independent practice associations have been particularly influential in building strong linkages between GPs and their communities in rural Maori areas and deprived inner city areas. Barnett and Barnett (1997) report how this integration with community needs can extend towards the promotion of the community ownership of general practice.

Alongside independent practice associations, another development associated with the internal market for general medical services in New Zealand has been the emergence of entrepreneurial medicine (Kearns and Barnett 1992, 1997, Barnett and Kearns 1996). This form of medical practice can be defined as one that is strongly team based and vigorously advertised; the providers of care and the owners of the facilities from which care is provided may often also be separate. The phenomenon has been most marked in Auckland and was facilitated by the passing of the Commerce Act 1986, which allowed doctors to advertise in the same way as other businesses, and by a relaxation of attitudes to advertising on the part of the New Zealand Medical Association. Early initiatives failed to thrive, but entrepreneurial medicine has subsequently 'made a distinct impact on the landscapes of New Zealand's larger cities' (Kearns and Barnett 1997:175). The particular focus has been on addressing the misuse of accident and emergency departments as primary care and on the provision of out-of-hours care. There has also been a marked tendency to offer discounted services. Two important consequences can be noted. First, entrepreneurial medicine has provided a basis for the emergence of the salaried GP as a counterpoint to the now general contractor model. This has in turn resulted in suggestions that the role of the GP in New Zealand is becoming more 'proletarianised' (McKinlay and Stoekle 1988, Barnett *et al.* 1998; see also Chapter 1). Second, it has forced some 'traditional' GPs into providing out-of-hours care in order to compete.

New Zealand came later to the internal market in health care than the UK, although, arguably, it came to it less abruptly. While there are substantial differences in general practice between the two countries, there are also points of similarity, and the transferability of initiatives has been high. Primary care was incorporated into the internal market somewhat more effectively and somewhat earlier in New Zealand, and, notwithstanding the differences resulting from the quasi-private nature of general practice in New

Zealand, it is in this integration that the most important pointers for the UK lie. The key issues have been discussed in the previous two paragraphs. First, when faced with a purchaser–provider split, providers will collaborate and organise. The parallels between independent practitioner associations and locality consortia or Scottish local health care cooperatives are considerable (see Chapter 4). There are less clear parallels with English PCGs as the commissioning role is not present. The second key issue is the space that the internal market makes for non-standard approaches to the provision of general medical care. As will be seen later in this chapter, entrepreneurial medicine is not without its parallels in the UK.

The USA – HMOs

As Kirkman-Liff (1997:30) asserts, 'the concept of the primary care physician is alien to the US; gatekeeping is not widely practised and there is an expectation of direct access to specialists'. Why then consider the USA? The short answer is that the USA is the stereotype of a free-market health care system, although it would be going a little far to term health care in the USA anything approaching a 'system', and the UK internal market represents a form of limited engagement with the notion that a market in health care can promote competition, which in turn can enhance efficiency. As a consequence, it is to the USA that it is appropriate to look for ideas about the management of the market for primary care. The influence of US ideas on the initial formulation of the UK internal market has been well documented (Enthoven 1985), and there can be no doubt that that influence continues to be potent. In the context of primary care, Chapter 4 characterised primary care groups as Britain's equivalent of US HMOs. Luft (1994), van de Ven *et al.* (1994) and Fairfield *et al.* (1997) all suggest that managed care, of which the HMO is a key form, is a probable model for the future organisation of health care systems. It is certainly an approach that is being increasingly implemented across Europe and not least, albeit with significant variations, in the UK. It is this parallel that this section will explore.

Managed care seeks to cut the costs of health care while maintaining its quality. Weiner and De Lissovoy (1993) have described the many different types of managed care structure as an 'unintelligible alphabet soup'. In the case of HMOs, individuals subscribe on the basis of an insurance premium, usually payable annually. The HMO arranges care when a subscriber becomes ill. The HMO is therefore a prepaid organised delivery system in which a fixed amount of funding is made available to cover the health needs of members. Le Grand (1998) suggests that managed care institutions such as HMOs now cover half of the insured population. HMOs essentially take on the financial risk associated with the potential costs of an individual's ill-health. They compete for custom by offering attractive packages of care and use community-based physicians as gatekeepers to specialised services. In this way, HMOs attempt to reduce the use and cost of secondary care. Community-based physicians are also themselves micro-managed (Fairfield *et al.* 1997) by the HMOs to ensure that they contain costs and improve quality. This is achieved by financial incentives, by profiling patterns of service use or by full or partial risk-adjusted capitation funding. The parallel with primary care groups is thus appropriate but partial. The HMO is a purchaser of primary and secondary care, but HMOs exist in a competitive environment whereas primary care groups do not.

Fairfield *et al.* (1997) discern three basic types of HMO. In the staff model, the HMO directly employs the physicians. In the context of primary care, these are unlikely to be generalists; instead they will be specialists with community-based offices. In the group model, community-based physicians organise as independent groups and work with the HMO on a contract basis, providing exclusive services to the subscribers to the HMO. Under the network model, it is the HMO that creates and facilitates the grouping of practices. Again, physician and HMO work together on a contract basis. In this model, the control that the HMO exerts over community-based physicians is far greater than that in the group model. In all models, subscribers to an HMO must choose a community-based physician recognised by the HMO. That physician then acts as a gatekeeper to specialist services. Recognised community-based physicians typically retain the right to provide services for several HMOs or to fee-for-service patients, or both. The network model is currently the fastest growing form of HMO. It represents a compromise between physician and HMO requirements and offers patients a wider selection of physicians. Network HMOs provide health care to some 35 million Americans.

The rise of the HMO in the USA has been a chequered one. Although the key rationale was cost containment, HMOs had little impact on health care costs until the mid-1980s (Salmon 1985). Indeed, the financial health of many HMOs themselves was often weak, and several were taken over or failed during the 1980s (Raffel and Raffel 1994). There was also substantial resistance from both the medical profession, for whom HMOs represented a threat to potential profits and medical autonomy, and patients, who were reluctant to be confined to recognised community-based physicians when choosing their doctors.

In equity terms, the verdict is also mixed. For Petchey (1987), US HMOs tended to underprovide for the poor and chronically sick, and 'cream-skim' the less costly patients from the local patient base. These issues raise clear parallels with those in the UK. These include the persistent allegations that GP fundholding practices also 'cream-skimmed' financially less burdensome potential patients and the perceptions that PCGs threaten the autonomy of

GPs. More broadly, the questionable financial effectiveness of HMOs during their development phase raises worries concerning the relative lack of economic evaluation of managed care initiatives in the UK.

A hallmark of HMO development in the USA has been the importance attached to the monitoring of community-based physician activity and the direction of that activity through the provision of clinical guidelines. Here too there are important parallels with the UK as both of these tasks are generally carried out by non-medical managers, even though clinical guidelines are usually authored by doctors. At issue is the extent to which medical activity is controlled and monitored by non-medical personnel. The basic idea is that potentially expensive decisions by community-based physicians should be subject to 'utilisation management' to ensure that they accord with guidelines and to allow the anticipation of probable costs. An analogy can be drawn with the health authority authorisation of extracontractual referrals in the early years of the internal market in the UK. Thus, important types of utilisation management are the precertification of inpatient admission, second-opinion programmes and the substitution of less expensive care whenever possible. With guidelines, the parallel is with the rapid emergence in Britain of evidence-based health care (Silagy and Haines 1998).

As Le Grand (1998) remarks, the (UK) NHS is rather successful at holding down costs. As many US HMOs are now developing systems for capitation payment and primary care gatekeeping that owe much to those of the UK in an effort to contain the still burgeoning costs of the US health care system, it might be thought that the lessons to be learnt from the US experience of HMOs are decreasing. Robinson and Steiner (1998), however, in what is perhaps the most comprehensive account of US-managed care, argue differently. They suggest that HMOs with the tightest organisation were able to achieve the greatest impact on community-based physician performance. These HMOs saw higher screening rates, more cost-consciousness and improved (or at least maintained) quality of care. Their contracted doctors had less variability in their practice styles and in their referral patterns. This, they argue, has clear consequences for PCGs in the UK as it indicates the importance of control. They also note that attempts by PCGs to benefit from this conclusion will not be popular. Any such attempts will challenge clinical autonomy and bring bureaucratic burdens for GPs that will be less than welcome.

The Netherlands

The Netherlands provides the third case study for the comparative section of this chapter. Like the UK, the Netherlands underwent a period of health policy reform in the late 1980s, which has continued to reverberate through the 1990s (van de Ven 1997). It was also one of the countries that influenced the reforms in New Zealand (Cumming and Salmond 1998). Unlike those of the UK or New Zealand, however, the reforms in the Netherlands have been delayed, adjusted and much diluted by the passage of time. The original vision of change has not been operationalised, notwithstanding the fact that Robinson (1998) suggests that the Dutch reform proposals represented the best compromise between the equity goal of universal access and the supposed efficiency of markets. The case study thus demonstrates the way in which change in the general practice arena can be both incremental and accomplished as a byproduct of intended rather than actual reform.

As was noted in Chapter 1, the Netherlands provides what is, in most respects, the nearest equivalent in the rest of Europe to the UK system of general practice. There is a substantial network of primary care provision, including some 7,000 GPs working as independent contractors and gate-keepers of access to secondary care (Okma 1995). The model of the independent contractor is essentially that of the UK save that, rather than contracting with a health authority, the GPs contract with a health insurance sickness fund. This difference reflects the contrasted funding bases of the two health services: a tax-funded national health service in the UK and a Bismarckian health insurance system in the Netherlands. In contrast to the UK situation, most Dutch GPs work in single-handed practices. Patients can choose their GP, and the GPs are paid on a capitation basis for poorer patients through the compulsory state health insurance system. Richer patients pay directly for services and are reimbursed by private health insurance.

In the mid-1980s, the health care system of the Netherlands was characterised as one based on government-regulated cartels in which GPs and the individual sickness funds were closely linked (van de Ven and Schut 1995). This did not provide for the most effective cost control, nor was it particularly efficient. Incentives and coordination were lacking. Although the basic state health insurance was centrally collected and then held by a central sickness funds council, the role of that council was simply to distribute funding to the separate individual sickness funds with which people had enrolled and who paid the GPs providers. Even though the number of sickness funds reduced through the 1980s, it could also be argued that the system was rather fragmented (van de Ven and Rutten 1994), particularly when considered in the additional context of some 40 private insurance firms servicing the health needs of richer people.

The 1987/88 reform proposals sought to rationalise this system. There were two main elements to what became known, after its chief proponent, as the Dekker plan. First there was to be compulsory risk-adjusted health insurance for all (de Roo 1995). Second, there was to be competition between insurance concerns (both the public sickness funds and the private firms) and between providers of health care. This plan metamorphosed into the Simons plan with a change of government and was scheduled for implementation first in 1992 and then in 1994. By 1994, as the government shifted to the left, it appeared that any comprehensive implementation of the Dekker–Simons reforms was unlikely (Robinson 1998). The 1995 Borst plan abandoned the objective of comprehensive basic insurance and shifted its focus onto the introduction of incentives. Managed competition was, however, retained.

In practice, therefore, it is the competition elements of the Dekker–Simons proposals that are important for the evolving shape of primary care in the Netherlands. The movement from cartels to competition has of course not been easy. Nor has it been welcomed, either by the insurance companies and sickness funds, or by the GPs. Nevertheless, clear legacies of Dekker can be found in the health care system as it presently operates. From 1992, GPs have been free to practise where they want; previously, they had to be licensed by a municipality. Sickness funds can now choose which GPs they contract with; previously they had to contract with any GP (Schut and van Doorslaer 1999). They are also allowed to vary the contracts that they put in place with GPs. Finally, although insurers have to provide a defined basic health care insurance package, they are permitted to offer extras benefits (van de Ven and Schut 1995). This development leads to a situation analogous to HMOs offering different service packages and promotes competition between sickness funds and patient choice.

For the UK, the most relevant of these developments is the choice now afforded to the sickness funds regarding the GPs with whom they work. If a PCG is seen as an NHS equivalent of a sickness fund, purchasing care not for its enrollees but for residents of its area, there might be two implications if the Dutch developments were applied in the UK context. First, PCGs or their successor PCTs might, subject of course to the necessary and not insubstantial legislative developments, seek to offer differentiated contracts to GPs. This might take the form of a different contract in each PCG; more radically, it might involve individual GP-specific contracts. Such a development would fundamentally challenge the notion of a national GP contract. Second, a PCG might choose to 'de-recognise' a GP who did not perform within defined parameters. This would enable a far greater regulation and control of practices within the primary care sector. It would also threaten the much-cherished independence and autonomy of UK GPs.

UK Futures

Dixon *et al.* (1998) underline the point made in Chapter 1 that, in the UK today, general practice is central to the operation of the NHS. In a primary care-led NHS, GPs have a major role. Although always important for the public, GPs have now lost their marginal position in the NHS and assumed centre stage. In this section, attention turns to an analysis of recent developments in the UK and the extent to which they presage a future for general practice that accentuates this increased visibility or one which may see a newly gained prominence lost as the wheels of change grind further forward.

GPs and Health Care Purchasing

In recent years, GPs' influence has particularly increased through their involvement in commissioning health care. The NHS reforms of 1991 encouraged GPs to influence health authorities via locality commissioning and impact directly on secondary care through the GP fundholding scheme (see Chapter 4). Total purchasing (Mays *et al.* 1997) gave GPs the opportunity to influence secondary care providers even more directly through the purchase of all hospital and community services rather than only those included in the standard fundholding scheme. Around 55 per cent of people in Britain were eventually registered with general practices operating some kind of fundholding scheme (Scottish Office Department of Health 1997), yet there was much variation in the detail of the ways in which GPs participated in these schemes – and they remained voluntary.

For Ham (1999), PCGs are an opportunity to build in a more structured and non-voluntary way on the achievements of general practice over the past 50 years. Their advent has, however, precipitated considerable confusion. On the one hand, politically and managerially orientated GPs have seized the chance to exert greater control over the resources available to PCGs and have relished the possibility of proceeding to PCT status and managing community services and community hospitals. On the other hand, there have been extensive debates over matters of control and clinical autonomy. GPs have veered between a determination to control PCGs and a desire to play as small a part as possible. They have, in particular, been much exercised by a realisation that PCTs will fall under the supervision of a lay majority board overseeing an executive with a professional (but not necessarily GP) majority. This is seen clearly as a threat to the autonomy of GPs and to their perceived perception of themselves as first among equals, if not first among a long list of also-rans, among community-based health professionals.

As will also be noted below, there are additional worries that PCGs and PCTs will precipitate a shift to a salaried status for GPs. Present indications are that independent contractor status will be safeguarded, but, in a way analogous to that pioneered in the LIZ initiative (see Chapter 7), flexible powers will be put in place to provide more opportunities for alternative employment models. Basic to all these potential threats to the newly emerged status of general practice is the cultural divide that separates the small business attitudes of GPs from the broader scale management concerns of PCGs. Managed care demands frameworks of accountability, clinical governance and regulation that sit ill with a profession with a tradition of antipathy to bureaucracy. As the Audit Commission (1999) argued in its review of the initial progress of PCGs, there is a need fully to engage all partners if PCGs are to succeed. This must include GPs.

Primary Care Act Pilots

Alhough the current salience of general practice in the UK may owe much to the role of GPs in the care commissioning process, it is as providers of care that they are best known to the public. Attention now turns to a number of developments that are currently challenging the traditional conception of GPs as the major public sector provider of primary medical care. The first such development concerns the measures promoted by the Primary Care Act 1997. This Act, squeezed through in the final weeks of the 1992 Major government, allowed NHS trusts to employ GPs directly and also develop other innovative ways of providing primary health care (Coulter and Mays 1997, Gillam 1999). General practice can now be provided under a contract made by health authorities with a NHS trust or group of practitioners instead of having to be provided by an independent contractor. In this style of practice, patients will register with the trust rather than with an individual doctor. The employed doctors will have contractual responsibilities to their employers.

Proposals were invited to pilot these new arrangements. After a selection process, 94 'personal medical services pilots' began in April 1998. By agreeing to provide personal medical services under Part I rather than Part II of the NHS Act 1977, GPs cease to be independent contractors. The chief impacts of this development are therefore to facilitate the further emergence of the salaried GP, to further challenge the status of independent contractor and to put in place an official alternative to employment under the 1990 GP contract. There appears to have been little generalised opposition from GPs to this development, although there has been some disquiet from local medical committees when NHS community trusts have sought to employ salaried GPs. Several practices used the scheme to develop shared management structures by contracting with intermediate organisations that provided such services (Gillam 1999). Thirty-three schemes based on community trusts were set up on the lines of the LIZ to address the needs of priority groups in deprived areas. Other schemes have been nurse led. Essentially, therefore, personal medical services pilots have been flexible and manyfold; they provide a basis for innovation in the provision arena.

Private General Practice

Goss (1998) rightly points out that UK GPs have always held multiple contracts alongside their main work as independent contractors to the NHS; GPs' very independence has allowed this and was designed to allow this. The collection of contracts and fee-for-service arrangements will include forensic medical work for the local police, occupational health services for local businesses and insurance certification. After the advent of the NHS, many GPs also retained a number of private patients who wished to pay the full cost of their care, often in anticipation of receiving better care, or who were covered by some form of private or mutual society health insurance. Goss's thesis is that, after the NHS was established, GPs became dependent on it for income but that the NHS is now, for a variety of both internal and external reasons, not adequate on its own as an income base for general practice.

Previous chapters have documented GPs' dissatisfaction with the 1990 contract, the bureaucratic burdens that it brought and the threat it posed to GP incomes. The advent of the 1990 contract needs to be seen alongside GP expectations of a high income as a reward for lengthy training and the tradition of GP autonomy. For those committed to remaining largely within the NHS, there is an increasing recognition of the personal and professional limits of GPs' ability to meet the patient and service demands resulting from the NHS reforms and the development of the primary care-led NHS. Some have been keen to take additional training to contract for non-core tasks or pursue careers that offer less direct patient care and more practice management. For others, seeking to enhance income and retain a maximal autonomy, there are attractions to be found in non-NHS activity. This activity might include commercial deputising services as well as private practice, or care for more complex groups of patients under supplementary contracts.

While these pressures for a greater role for private general medical practice have not (yet) resulted in anything approaching New Zealand's entrepreneurial sector, there is little doubt that it is attractive to some GPs. Furthermore, there are important parallels in the progressive disappearance of free, or at least non-means tested, non-medical primary care that suggest that the public would acquiesce, if not accept, a rather larger non-NHS general medical sector. Clear evidence to this end comes from the lack of overt protest that accompanied the introduction of prescription charges and payment for optical services. The most obvious pointer for the future, however, is provided by the fate of NHS dental services. In the face of perceptions of income erosion and over-regulation, dentists, through the 1980s and 90s, increasingly pursued the exit option, left the NHS and moved into fee-for-service or insurance-based work. In many parts of the country, NHS dentistry has now become rare apart from in the form of salaried community dentists employed by NHS community trusts. Personal medical services pilots, of course, raise exactly that possibility for general medical practice should GPs decide in greater numbers to contract individually with private patients.

Walk-in Centres

Chapter 7 made much of the use of hospital accident and emergency departments as general medical care providers in urban areas. Earlier in the present chapter, the New Zealand experience with entrepreneurial walk-in clinics was reviewed. The impetus behind both initiatives was the fact that general medical care is not always available 'on tap' when it is needed. In spring 1999, it was announced that 20 walk-in NHS medical centres would be set up to address this problem (Ham 1999). A sum of £280m was set aside for these 20 pilot centres to be run directly by PCGs. The prime role of the walk-in centres was to offer quick and convenient treatment. They also included out-of-hours cover and, in some areas, a 'one-stop service' additionally incorporating social work and community psychiatric nursing. Notably, in terms of parallels with other developments, they were to employ salaried GPs alongside the extensive use of nurse practitioners.

At the present stage, it is too early to offer any considered evaluation of walk-in centres. Certainly, albeit to a minor extent at present, they offer the possibility of bypassing GPs and subverting the traditional GP gatekeeper role. They also provide a further challenge to the independent contractor status. Ham (1999) suggests that it is debatable whether they are an appropriate response to the desire to improve access to services. The pilot scheme possibly has too few centres to make a reasoned judgement on this issue, and comparison should be made with less radical measures of demand management. Ham also notes the unclear relationship between the walk-in centres and the personal medical services pilots and raises the spectre of 'initiative fatigue' hitting the primary medical care arena. His conclusion is perhaps closest to the truth: 'given the almost universal admiration of British general practice, and evidence that it is highly valued by patients, ad hoc developments like walk in centres appear to be directed as much at the spin doctors as their medical counterparts' (Ham 1999:1092).

It is, however, not only New Labour who have seized upon walk-in clinics as a possible solution to the access problems of general medicine. Private primary care walk-in centres also emerged in 1999. McIntosh (1999) discusses the rise of the Medicentre chain of private walk-in clinics based in large retail outlets, most notably the Sainsburys chain of food stores. The Medicentre chain is strongly reminiscent of New Zealand entrepreneurial medicine in seeking to provide on-the-spot, check-up-type health care for people on constrained time budgets. Run by Sinclair Montrose Health Care, the chain offered (as of April 1999) 11 clinics located in suburban London shopping malls (six) and similar locations in the West Midlands, Sheffield and Gateshead. Business consisted of corporate health checks as well as some 100 walk-in patients per week at each branch.

NHS Direct

The final initiative to be discussed in this section is NHS Direct. NHS Direct is a telephone triage system operated by nurses to advise callers on the most appropriate form of care. It is, like walk-in centres, intended to provide an alternative, more accessible form of health care consultation. Florin and Rosen (1999) see it in the context of the information revolution and the rise of the virtual society. While the traditional GP consultation has undoubted value, contemporary technology and, more importantly, patients' familiarity with that technology is such that a well-trained practitioner, with appropriate decision-making support, could come close to replicating the effectiveness of the GP consultation – at a fraction of the cost.

Munro *et al.* (1998) provide a preliminary evaluation of NHS Direct. Their conclusions are mixed. Call rates were two-thirds lower than expected over the first eight months of operation and varied sixfold between the three pilot areas (Lancashire, Milton Keynes and Northumbria). The service was essentially used for out-of-hours advice rather than as a substitute for a GP visit. Users fitted closely to the standard demographics of GP attenders with one important exception: older people, a major user group for GP services, were under-represented. The availability of the service had no significant effect on approaches to other services such as the ambulance service, accident and emergency departments or general practice. Finally, there were substantial differences in the advice given from each of the three centres regarding 120 identical dummy cases.

These results would seem to provide cause for some concern if NHS Direct is to be a major force in demand management in the primary care-led NHS. It may well be that, rather than providing a substitute layer of care management, it actually generates more work. A second concern is the issue of continuity of care. Munro *et al.* (1998) argue that advice is more likely to be appropriate if it is given by someone who knows a patient's history. While that knowledge may be present in a GP practice, it is unlikely to be held by NHS Direct. It would be possible to conclude that bypassing that knowledge in the interests of a technologically led solution to high demand may ultimately not only marginalise GPs, but also endanger patients. To this end, NHS Direct might function better as a source for information rather than a point of access for medical advice. This pessimistic view is, however, not shared by the government, which sees NHS Direct as a major element in future primary care demand management.

Conclusion

The key theme of this final chapter has been the challenge that now faces general practice in the UK. Chapman and Groom (1999) term this a move from a complex but stable environment to one characterised by complexity and instability. Lessons from abroad and emerging initiatives in the UK mean that general practice is likely to change radically over the next few years unless it is astonishingly forthright and conservative in protecting its present manifestation. Its very adaptability and flexibility, as evidenced in its history and particularly in its encounter with policy developments over the past decade, would suggest that it will metamorphose rather than resist. The preceding chapters have, at times, been critical. Overall, however, it must be concluded that UK general practice is indeed a major jewel in the NHS crown. It is paradoxical that, just as it has achieved a position of centrality within the NHS, it faces changes that challenge significantly its ability to maintain that position without itself changing significantly.

The major issue at stake is arguably independent contractor status. The 1990 GP contract ushered in an increasingly managed service, the Primary Care Act 1997 enabled alternative models of primary care and encouraged salaried options, and the probable emergence of PCTs raises the very real prospect of a shift from independent contractor status to salaried employment (Oldham and Rutter 1999). Many GPs now feel that their independence is increasingly illusory. Chapman and Groom (1999) provide an interesting and thoughtful summary of the issues involved. On the one hand, independent contractor status provides flat autonomous work structures. GP practices are also an effective size for responsive interaction with patients and enable innovation and flexibility. On the other hand, independent contractor status has sheltered some isolationism and poor practice. It may not suit all circumstances, all individuals or all parts of the UK. Crucially, there is a lack of evidence concerning why and how independent contractor status is crucial to (good) general practice. It is no longer a defining characteristic of general practice in the UK, even if it remains a revered symbol in a world in which, in the words of John Chisholm, chairman of the BMA General Practitioners' Committee (quoted in Beecham 1999): 'We need to take stock of what being a GP should mean in the next millennium, what we need from government, and what we expect of ourselves.'

Bibliography

ACHCEW (Association of Community Health Councils for England and Wales) (1986) *A Response to the Government Consultation on Primary Care*, London: ACHCEW.

Acheson, D. (1998) *Report of the Independent Inquiry into Inequalities in Health*, London: HMSO.

Agass, M., Coulter, A., Mant, J. and Fuller, A. (1991) Patient participation in general practice: who participates? *British Journal of General Practice*, **41**, 198–201.

Allen, D., Harley, M. and Makinson, G. (1987) Performance indicators in the National Health Service, *Social Policy and Administration*, **21**, 70–84.

Allsop, J. and May, A. (1986) *The Emperor's New Clothes: Family Practitioner Committees in the 1980s*, London: King's Fund.

Andalo, D. (1998) GP duties revealed for new NHS, *GP*, 10 April, 3.

Armstrong, D. (1979) The emancipation of biographical medicine, *Social Science and Medicine*, **13A**, 1–8.

Armstrong, D. (1985) Space and time in British general practice, *Social Science and Medicine*, **20**, 659–66.

Armstrong, D., Granville, T., Bailey, E. and O'Keefe, G. (1990) Doctor-initiated consultations: a study of communication between general practitioners and patients about the need for re-attendance, *British Journal of General Practice*, **40**, 241–2.

Armstrong, I. and Haston, W. (1997) Medical decision support for remote general practitioners using telemedicine, *Journal of Telemedicine and Telecare*, **3**, 27–34.

Audit Commission (1986) *Making a Reality of Community Care*, London: HMSO.

Audit Commission (1994) *A Prescription for Improvement. Towards More Rational Prescribing*, London: HMSO.

Audit Commission (1996) *What the Doctor Ordered. A Study of GP Fundholders in England and Wales*, London: HMSO.

Audit Commission (1999) *PCGs: An Early View of Primary Care Groups in England*, London: HMSO.

Baggott, R. (1994) *Health and Health Care in Britain*, Basingstoke: Macmillan.

Bain, J. (1990) Child health surveillance, *British Medical Journal*, **300**, 1381–2.

Balarajan, R., Yuen, P. and Machin, D. (1992) Deprivation and general practitioner workload, *British Medical Journal*, **304**, 529–34.

Balint, M. (1957, reprinted 1964) *The Doctor, His Patient and the Illness*, Tunbridge Wells: Pitman Medical.

Balogh, R. (1995) *Evaluation of Locality Planning in Northumberland*, Morpeth: Northumberland Health Authority.

Balogh, R. (1996) Exploring the role of localities in health commissioning: a review of the literature, *Social Policy and Administration*, **30**(2), 99–113.

Barnard, K., Lee, K., Mills, A. and Reynolds, J. (1980) NHS Planning: an assessment, *Hospital and Health Services Review*, August, 262–5.

Barnett, P. and Barnett, R. (1997) A turning tide? Reflections on ideology and health service restructuring in New Zealand, *Health and Place*, **3**, 55–8.

Barnett, R. and Kearns, R. (1996) Shopping around? Consumerism and the use of private accident and emergency clinics in Auckland, New Zealand, *Environment and Planning A*, **28**, 1053–75.

Barnett, R., Barnett, P. and Kearns, R. (1998) Declining professional dominance? Trends in the proletarianisation of primary care in New Zealand, *Social Science and Medicine*, **46**, 197–207.

Bartlett, W. (1996) The regulation of general practice in the UK, *International Journal of Health Planning and Management*, **11**(3), 3–18.

Beecham, L. (1999) UK GPs will produce blueprint for the future, *British Medical Journal*, **319**, 12.

Bentham, G. and Haynes, R. (1992) Evaluation of a mobile branch surgery in a rural area, *Social Science and Medicine*, **34**, 97–102.

Benzeval, M. and Judge, K. (1996) Access to health care in England: continuing inequalities in the distribution of GPs, *Journal of Public Health Medicine*, **18**, 33–40.

Benzeval, M., Judge, K. and New, B. (1991) Health and health care in London, *Public Money and Management*, **11**, 25–32.

Berwick, D., Enthoven, A. and Bunker, J. (1992) Quality management in the NHS: the doctor's role, *British Medical Journal*, **304**, 235–9.

Bhopal, R. and Samin, A. (1988) Immunisation uptake of Glasgow Asian children: benefits of the communication barrier, *Community Medicine*, **10**, 215–20.

Bhopal, R. S., Moffat, S., Pless Mullorr, T., Phillimore, B. R. *et al.* (1998) Does living near a constellation of petrochemical, steel, and other industries impair health? *Occupational and Environmental Medicine*, **55**(12), 812–22.

Billingshurst, B. and Whitfield, M. (1993) Why do patients change their general practitioner? A postal questionnaire study of patients in Avon, *British Journal of General Practice*, **43**, 336–8.

Birchall, E. (1992) *Working Together in Child Protection: Report of Phase Two, A Survey of the Experience and Perceptions of Six Key Professions*, Stirling: University of Stirling.

Birchall, E. (1995) Child protection. In P. Owens, J. Carrier and J. Horder (eds) *Interprofessional Issues in Community and Primary Health Care*, London: Macmillan.

Blaxter, M. (1990) *Health and Lifestyles*, London: Tavistock.

BMA (British Medical Association) (1995a) *Survey on the Impact of the Implementation of the Community Care Reforms: General Practitioners*, London: Health Policy and Economic Research Unit, British Medical Association.

BMA (British Medical Association) (1995b) *Core Values for the Medical Profession in the 21st Century*, Survey Report, London: British Medical Association.

BMA (British Medical Association) (1997) *Medical Involvement in the Commissioning Process: A Report of a National Study of Health Authorities and LMCs in England*, London: Health Policy and Economic Research Unit, British Medical Association.

Boerma, W., Groenewegen, P. and Van der Zee, J. (1998) General practice in urban and rural Europe: the range of curative services, *Social Science and Medicine*, **47**, 445–53.

Bond, J., Cartilidge, A., Gregson, B., Philips, P., Bolam, F. and Gill, K. (1985) *A Study of Interprofessional Collaboration in Primary Health Care Organisations*, Report No. 27, Vol. 2, Newcastle upon Tyne: Health Care Research Unit, University of Newcastle.

Bosanquet, N. and Salisbury, C. (1998) The practice. In I. Loudon, J. Horder and C. Webster (eds) *General Practice under the National Health Service 1948–1997*, London: Clarendon.

Bowling, A., Farqhuar, M. and Browne, P. (1991) Use of services in old age: data from three surveys of elderly people, *Social Science and Medicine*, **33**, 689–700.

Boyle, S. and Smaje, C. (1992) Minor surgery in general practice: the effect of the 1990 GP contract. In A. Harrison (ed.) *Health Care UK 1991*, London: King's Fund.

Bradley, A. (1987) Poverty and dependency in village England. In P. Lowe, A. Bradley and S. Wright (eds) *Disadvantage and Welfare in Rural Areas*, Norwich: Geo Books.

Brand, J. (1965) *Doctors and the State*, Baltimore: Johns Hopkins Press.

Brown, K., Williams, E. and Groom, L. (1992) Health checks on patients 75 years and over in Nottinghamshire after the new GP contract, *British Medical Journal*, **305**, 619–21.

Bruce, N. and Burnett, S. (1991) Prevention of lifestyle-related disease: general practitioners' views about their role, effectiveness and resources, *Family Practitioner*, **8**, 373–7.

Bryce, C., Curtis, S. and Mohan, J. (1994) Coronary heart disease: trends in spatial inequalities and implications for health care planning in England, *Social Science and Medicine*, **38**, 677–90.

Buckingham, K. and Freeman, P. (1997) Sociodemographic and morbidity indicators of need in relation to the use of community health services: observational study, *British Medical Journal*, **315**, 994–6.

Buckley, M. (1997) Industrious resolution, *Health Service Journal*, **107**(5568), 32–3.

Butler, J. (1987) *Too Many Patients*, London: Avebury.

Butler, J. (1992) *Patients, Policies and Politics: Before and after Working for Patients*, Buckingham: Open University Press.

Butler, J., Bevan, J. and Taylor, R. (1973) *Family Doctors and Public Policy*, London: Routledge & Kegan Paul.

Calnan, M. and Butler, J. (1988) The economy of time in general practice: an estimate of the influence of list size, *Social Science and Medicine*, **26**, 435–551.

Calnan, M. and Gabe, J. (1991) Recent development in general practice. In J. Gabe, M. Calnan and M. Bury (eds) *The Sociology of the Health Service*, London: Routledge.

Calnan, M. and Hutten, J. (1992) Professional reimbursement and management of time in general practice, *Social Science and Medicine*, **35**, 209–16.

Carlisle, R. and Johnstone, S. (1998) The relationship between census-derived socio-economic variables and general practice consultation rates in three town centre practices, *British Journal of General Practice*, **48**, 1675–8.

Carr-Hill, R. and Sheldon, T. (1991) Designing a deprivation payment for general practitioners: the UPA(8) wonderland, *British Medical Journal*, **302**, 393–6.

Carr-Hill, R., Rice, N. and Roland, M. (1996) Socioeconomic determinants of rates of consultation in general practice based on the fourth national morbidity survey of general practices, *British Medical Journal*, **312**, 1008–12.

Cartwright, A. (1967) *Patients and Their Doctors*, London: Routledge & Kegan Paul.

Cartwright, A. and Anderson, R. (1981) *General Practice Revisited: A Second Study of Patients and Their Doctors*, London: Tavistock.

Cartwright, A. and O'Brien, M. (1976) Social class variations in health care and in the nature of general practice consulations. In M. Stacey (ed.) *Sociological Review Monograph*, **22**, Keele: University of Keele.

Casey, P. and Tyrer, P. (1990) Personality disorder and psychiatric illness in general practice, *British Journal of Psychiatry*, **156**, 261–5.

Central Statistical Office (1994) *Social Trends*, London: HMSO.

Chambers, R. and Belcher, J. (1993) Work patterns of general practitioners before and after the introduction of the 1990 contract, *British Journal of General Practice*, **43**, 410–12.

Chapman, R. and Groom, H. (1999) For and against: should we fight to preserve the independent contractor status of general practitioners? *British Medical Journal*, **318**, 797–8.

Charlton, J. and Lakhani, A. (1985) Is the Jarman underprivileged area score valid? *British Medical Journal*, **290**, 1714–16.

Cherry, S. (1996) *Medical Services and the Hospitals in Britain, 1860–1939*, Cambridge: Cambridge University Press.

Chisholm, J. (1990) The 1990 contract: its history and its content, *British Medical Journal*, **300**, 853–6.

Chisholm, J. (1998) Primary care and the NHS white papers, *British Medical Journal*, **316**, 1687–8.

Cleary, P. (1999) The increasing importance of patient surveys, *British Medical Journal*, **319**, 720–1.

Committee of Inquiry (1974) *Report of the Inquiry into the Care and Supervision Provided in Relation to Maria Colwell*, London: HMSO.

Corney, R. (1995) Mental health services. In P. Owens, J. Carrier and J. Horder (eds) *Interprofessional Issues in Community and Primary Health Care*, London: Macmillan.

Cotgrove, A., Bell, G. and Katona, C. (1992) Psychiatric admissions and social deprivation: is the Jarman underprivileged area score relevant? *Journal of Epidemiology and Community Health*, **46**, 245–7.

Coulter, A. (1995) Evaluating general practitioner fundholding in the United Kingdom, *European Journal of Public Health*, **5**, 1–13.

Coulter, A. (1999) Paternalism or partnership? *British Medical Journal*, **319**, 719–20.

Coulter, A. and Bradlaw, J. (1993) Effect of NHS reforms on general practitioners' referral patterns, *British Medical Journal*, **306**, 433–7.

Coulter, A. and Mays, N. (1997) Deregulating primary care, *British Medical Journal*, **314**, 510–13.

Coulter, A. and Schofield, T. (1991) Prevention in general practice: the views of doctors in the Oxford region, *British Journal of General Practice*, **41**, 140–3.

Cox, J. (ed.) (1995) *Rural General Practice in the United Kingdom*, RCGP Occasional Paper No. 71, London: Royal College of General Practitioners.

Cox, J. (1998) Poverty in rural areas, *British Medical Journal*, **316**, 722–30.

Cule, J. (1980) *A Doctor for the People*, London: Update.

Cumming, J. and Salmond, G. (1998) Reforming New Zealand health care. In W. Ranade (ed.) *Markets and Health Care: A Comparative Analysis*, London: Longman.

Curtis, S. (1987) The patient's view of general practice in an urban area, *Family Practice*, **4**, 200–6.

Curtis, S. (1990) Use of survey data and small area statistics to assess the link between individual morbidity and neighbourhood deprivation, *Journal of Epidemiology and Community Health*, **44**, 62–8.

Curtis, S. and Taket, A. (1997) *Health and Societies: Changing Perspectives*, London: Arnold.

Dalley, G. (1991) Beliefs and behaviour: professionals and the policy process, *Journal of Aging Studies*, **5**(2), 163–80.

Davies, B. (1968) *Social Needs and Resources in Local Services*, London: Michael Joseph.

Dawson, A. (1996) Supporting secondary care transfers. In G. Meads (ed.) *A Primary Care-led NHS*, London: Churchill Livingstone.

Day, P. and Klein, R. (1987) *Accountabilities Five Public Services*, Tavistock: London.

De Roo, A. (1995) Contracting and solidarity: market-oriented changes in Dutch health insurance schemes. In R. Saltman and C. Von Otter (eds) *Implementing Planned Markets in Health Care*, Buckingham: Open University Press.

DHSS (Department of Health and Social Security) (1976a) *Prevention and Health: Everybody's Business*, London: HMSO.

DHSS (Department of Health and Social Security) (1976b) *Sharing Resources for Health in England*, London: HMSO.

DHSS (Department of Health and Social Security) (1977) *Prevention and Health*, London: HMSO.

DHSS (Department of Health and Social Security) (1980) *Inequalities in Health*, (Black Report), London: DHSS.

DHSS (Department of Health and Social Security) (1981a) *The Primary Care Team*, Report of a Joint Working Group of the Standard Medical Advisory Committee and the Standard Nursing and Midwifery Committee, chaired by Dr W.G. Harding, London: HMSO.

DHSS (Department of Health and Social Security) (1981b) *Care in Action: Consultative Document*, London: HMSO.

DHSS (Department of Health and Social Security) (1983) *NHS Management Inquiry*, (Griffiths Management Report), London: HMSO.

DHSS (1986a) (Cumberlege Report). *Neighbourhood Nursing – A Focus for Care*, Report of the Community Nursing Review, London: HMSO.

DHSS (Department of Health and Social Security) (1986b) *Primary Health Care: An Agenda for Discussion*, Cmnd 9771, London: HMSO.

DHSS (Department of Health and Social Security) (1987) *Promoting Better Health: the Government's Programme for Improving Primary Health Care*, Cmnd 249, London: HMSO.

DHSS (Department of Health and Social Security) (1988) *Community Care: An Agenda for Action*, (The Griffiths Community Care Report), London: HMSO.

DHSS (Department of Health and Social Security) (NI) (1998) *Fit for the Future: the Government's Proposals for the Future of the Health and Personal Social Services in Northern Ireland*, Belfast: DHSS.

Dixon, J., Holland, P. and Mays, N. (1998) Primary care core values: developing primary care: gatekeeping, commissioning, and managed care, *British Medical Journal*, **317**, 125–8.

Dixon M., Murray, T. and Jenner, D. (1997) *The Locality Commissioning Handbook: From Vision to Reality*, Oxford: Radcliffe Medical Press.

DoH (Department of Health) (1989a) *Working for Patients*, Cm 555, London: HMSO.

DoH (Department of Health) (1989b) *Caring for People: Community Care in the Next Decade and Beyond*, Cm 849, London: HMSO.

DoH (Department of Health) (1990) *Working for Patients: Guidance for Family Health Services*, London: HMSO.

DoH (Department of Health) (1992a) *The Health of the Nation*, London: HMSO.

DoH (Department of Health) (1992b) *On the State of the Public Health*, London: HMSO.

DoH (Department of Health) (1992c) *Report of the Inquiry into London's Health Service, Medical Education and Research* (Tomlinson Report), London: HMSO.

DoH (Department of Health) (1993) *Making London Better*, London: HMSO.

DoH (Department of Health) (1994) *Being Heard: The Report of a Committee on NHS Complaints Procedures*, London: HMSO.

DoH (Department of Health) (1995) *Acting on Complaints: The Government's Proposals in Response to Being Heard*, London: HMSO.

DoH (Department of Health) (1996a) *Primary Care: Delivering the Future*, London: HMSO.

DoH (Department of Health) (1996b) *Choice and Opportunity: Primary Care – the Future*, London: HMSO.

DoH (Department of Health) (1997) *The New NHS: Modern, Dependable*, Cm 3807, London: Stationery Office.

DoH (Department of Health) (1998a) *Partnership in Action (New Opportunities for Joint Working between Health and Social Services): A Discussion Document*, London: DoH.

DoH (Department of Health) (1998b) *A First Class Service*, London: DoH.

DoH (Department of Health) (1998c) *Statistics for General Medical Practitioners in England: 1987–1997*, Bulletin 1998/16, London: DoH.

DoH (Department of Health)/Welsh Office (1989) *General Practice in the National Health Service. A New Contract*, London, Stationery Office.

DoH (Department of Health)/Welsh Office (1998) *NHS Wales: Putting Patients First*, London: Stationery Office.

Dolan, S., Jarman, B., Bajekal, M., Davies, P. and Hart, D. (1995) Measuring disadvantage: changes in the underprivileged area, Townsend, and Carstairs scores 1981–91, *Journal of Epidemiology and Community Health*, **49** (Supplement 2), S30–S33.

Dowling, B. (1997) Effect of fundholding on waiting list times: database study, *British Medical Journal*, **315**, 290–2.

Eames, M., Ben-Shlomo, Y. and Marmot, M. (1992) Social deprivation and premature mortality: regional comparison across England, *British Medical Journal*, **307**, 1097–102.

Eaton, L. (1997) Vital signs are poor, *Community Care*, 17–23 April, 18–19.

Eckstein, H. (1958) *The English Health Service*, Cambridge, MA: Harvard University Press.

Elston, M. (1991) The politics of professional power: medicine in a changing health service. In J. Gabe, M. Calnan and M. Bury (eds) *The Sociology of the Health Service*, London: Routledge.

Emanuel, E. and Emanuel, L. (1996) What is accountability in health care? *Annals of Internal Medicine*, **124**, 229–39.

Enthoven, A. (1985) *Reflections on the Management of the NHS*, London: Nuffield Provincial Hospitals Trust.

Fairfield, G., Hunter, D., Dubos, R. and Rosleff, F. (1997) Managed care: origins, principles, and evolution, *British Medical Journal*, **314**, 1823.

Fearn, R. (1983) The role of the branch surgery in accessibility to primary health care in rural Norfolk, unpublished PhD thesis, Norwich: University of East Anglia.

Fearn, R., Haynes, R. and Bentham, G. (1984) The role of branch surgeries in a rural area, *Journal of Royal College of General Practitioners*, **34**, 488–91.

Fitzpatrick, R. (1984) Satisfaction with health care. In R. Fitzpatrick, J. Hinton, S. Newton, G. Scambler and J. Thompson (eds) *The Experience of Illness*, London: Tavistock.

Florin, D. and Rosen, R. (1999) Evaluating NHS direct, *British Medical Journal*, **319**, 5–6.

Forsyth, G. (1966) *Doctors and State Medicine. A Study of the British Health Service*, London: Pitman Medical.

Fougère, G. (1993) Struggling for control: the state and the medical profession in New Zealand. In F. Hafferty and J. McKinlay (eds) *The Changing Medical Profession*, Oxford: Oxford University Press.

Fox, A., Jones, D. and Goldblatt, P. (1984) Approaches to studying the effect of socio-economic circumstances on geographic differences in mortality in England and Wales, *British Medical Bulletin*, **40**, 309–14.

Freake, D., Crowley, P., Steiner, M. and Drinkwater, C. (1997) Local heroes, *Health Service Journal*, **107**(5561), 28–9.

Freeman, G. and Richards, S. (1990) How much personal care in four group practices, *British Medical Journal*, **301**, 1028-30.

Freeman, H. (1996) Stimulus for change – the evolution of fundholding. In P. Littlejohns and C. Victor (eds) *Making Sense of a Primary Care-led Health Service*, Oxford: Radcliffe Medical Press.

Freidson, E. (1970a) *Profession of Medicine: A Study of the Sociology of Applied Knowledge*, London: Harper & Row.

Freidson, E. (1970b) *Professional Dominance: The Social Structure of Medical Care*, New York: Atherton Press.

Fry, J. (1983) *Present State and Future Needs in General Practice*, Lancaster: MTP Press.

Fry, J. (1988) *General Practice and Primary Health Care*, London: Nuffield Provincial Hospitals Trust.

Fry, J. (1991) *General Practice: The Facts*, London: Nuffield Provincial Hospitals Trust.

Fry, J. and Horder, J. (1994) *Primary Care in an International Context*, London: Nuffield Provincial Hospitals Trust.

Gafni, A. (1999) Shared decision-making in a publicly funded health care system, *British Medical Journal*, **319**, 725–6.

Gamble, A. (1988) *The Free Economy and the Strong State: The Politics of Thatcherism*, London: Macmillan.

GB Departments of Health (1989) *General Practice in the National Health Service: The 1990 Contract*, London: HMSO.

Gibson, R. (1981) *The Family Doctor: His Life and History*, London: George Allen & Unwin.

Gibson, R. (1988) The fall and rise of general practice, *British Medical Journal*, **297**, 44–6.

Gillam, S. (1992) Provision of health promotion clinics in relation to population need: another example of the inverse care law? *British Journal of General Practice*, **42**, 54–6.

Gillam, S. (1999) Does the new NHS need personal medical services pilots? *British Medical Journal*, **318**, 1302–3.

Glendinning, C. and Lloyd, B. (1998) The continuing care guidelines and primary and community health services, *Health and Social Care in the Community*, **6**(3), 181–8.

Glennerster, H., Matsaganis, M., Owens, P. and Hancock, S. (1994) *Implementing GP Fundholding: Wild Card or Winning Hand?* Buckingham: Open University Press.

GMC (General Medical Council) (1998) *Good Medical Practice*, London: GMC.

GMS (General Medical Services) (1992) *The National Health Services for England and Wales Regulations*, London: HMSO.

GMSC (General Medical Services Committee) (1993) *The New Health Promotion Package*, London: BMA.

GMSC (General Medical Services Committee) (1996) *Core Services: Taking the Initiative*, London: BMA.

Godber, C. (1995) Reflections on a brief return to strategic planning. In F. Honigsbaum, J. Richards and T. Lockett (eds) *Priority Setting in Action*, Oxford: Radcliffe Medical Press.

Godber, G. (1975) *The Health Service: Past, Present and Future*, London: Athlone.

Gordon. P. and Hadley, J. (1996) *Extending Primary Care: Polyclinics, Resource Centres, Hospitals at Home*, Oxford: Radcliffe Medical Press.

Goss, B. (1998) Contracting for general practice: another turn of the wheel of history, *British Medical Journal*, **316**, 1953–5.

Graham, H. (1984) *Women, Health and the Family*, New York: Harvester Wheatsheaf.

Greagsby, P. and Milner, P. (1996) Combining with public health. In G. Meads (ed.) *A Primary Care-led NHS*, London: Churchill Livingstone.

Green, J. (1993) The views of singlehanded general practitioners: a qualitative study, *British Medical Journal*, **290**, 823–6.

Green, J. (1996) Time and space revisited: the creation of community in single-handed British general practice, *Health and Place*, **2**, 85–94.

Griffiths, C., Sturdy, P., Naish, J., Omar, R. *et al.* (1997) Hospital admissions for asthma in east London: associations with characteristics of local general practices, prescribing, and population, *British Medical Journal*, **314**, 482–6.

Groenwegen P., van der Zee, J. and van Haaften, R. (1991) *The Remuneration of General Practitioners in Western Europe*, London: Avebury.

Groves, T. (1999) Reforming British primary care (again), *British Medical Journal*, **318**, 747–8.

Ham, C. (1992a) *Health Policy in Britain*, Basingstoke: Macmillan.

Ham, C. (1992b) *Locality Purchasing*, Birmingham: Health Services Management Centre.

Ham, C. (1999) New Labour and the NHS, *British Medical Journal*, **318**, 1092.

Hancock, C. (1998) The long and winding road, *Nursing Times*, **94**(2), 24.

Hannay, D., Usherwood, T. and Platts, M. (1992) Workload of general practitioners before and after the new contract, *British Medical Journal*, **304**, 615–18.

Harris, C.M. and Scrivenor, G. (1996) Fundholders' prescribing costs: the first five years, *British Medical Journal*, **313**, 1531–4.

Harrison, R., Clayton, W. and Wallace, P. (1997) Is there a role for telemedicine in an urban environment? *Journal of Telemedicine and Telecare*, **3** (Supplement 1), 15–17.

Harrison, S. and Hunter, D. (1994) *Rationing Health Care*, London: Insitutute for Public Policy Research.

Harrison, S. and Pollitt, C. (1994) *Controlling Health Professionals: The Future of Work and Organisation in the NHS*, Buckingham: Open University Press.

Hasler, J. (1992) The primary health care team: history and contractual farces, *British Medical Journal*, **305**, 232–4.

Hasler, J. (1996) *The Primary Health Care Team*, London: Royal Society of Medicine.

Hasler, J., Hemphill, P.M.R., Stewart, T.I., Boyle, N. *et al.* (1968) Development of the nursing section of the community health team, *British Medical Journal*, **iii**, 734–6.

Hassell, K., Harris, J., Rogers, A., Noyce, P. and Wilkinson, J. (1996) *The Role and Contribution of Pharmacy in Primary Care*, Manchester: National Primary Care Research and Development Centre.

Hassell, K., Noyce, P., Rogers, A., Harris, J. and Wilkinson, J. (1997) A pathway to the GP: the pharmaceutical consultation as a first port of call in primary health care, *Family Practice*, **14**, 458–61.

Hayden, J. (1996) The importance of general practice in a primary care led National Health Service, *British Journal of General Practice*, May, 267–8.

Healy, P. (1997) Uneasy bedfellows, *Health Service Journal*, 6 November, 10–11.

Henwood, M. (1995) Strained relations, *Health Service Journal*, 6 July, 22–23.

Heritage, Z. (ed.) (1994) *Community Participation in Primary Care*, Occasional Paper No. 64, London: Royal College of General Practitioners.

Herity, B., McDonald, P., Johnson, Z. *et al.* (1997) A pilot study of cervical screening in an inner city area – lessons for a national programme, *Cytopathology*, **8**, 161–70

Higgins, R., Oldman, C. and Hunter, D. (1995) Working together: lessons for collaboration between health and social services, *Health and Social Care*, **2**, 269–77.

Hine, C. and Bachmann, M. (1997) What does locality commissioning in Avon offer? Retrospective descriptive evaluation, *British Medical Journal*, **314**, 1246–50.

Hippisley-Cox, J., Hardy, C., Pringle, M., Fielding, K., Carlisle, R. and Chilvers, C. (1997) The effect of deprivation on variations in general practitioners referral rates: a cross sectional study of computerised data on new medical and surgical outpatient referrals in Nottinghamshire, *British Medical Journal*, **314**, 1458–61.

Hirschman, A. (1970) *Exit, Voice and Loyalty: Responses to Decline in Firms, Organisations and States*, London: Harvard University Press.

Honigsbaum, F. (1979) *The Division in British Medicine. A History of the Separation of General Practice from Hospital Care 1911–1968*, London: Kogan Page.

Hopton, J. and Heaney, D. (1999) The development of local healthcare cooperatives in Scotland, *British Medical Journal*, **318**, 1185–7.

Horder, J. (1998) Developments in other countries. In I. Loudon, J. Horder and C. Webster (eds) *General Practice Under the National Health Service 1948–1997*, London: Clarendon Press.

Horrobin, G. and McIntosh, J. (1983) Time, risk and routine in general practice, *Sociology of Health and Illness*, **5**, 312–31.

Howie, J., Porter, A. and Forbes, J. (1989) Quality and the use of time in general practice, *British Medical Journal*, **298**, 1008–10.

Howie, J., Heaney, D. and Maxwell, M. (1995) Evaluating care of patients with selected health problems in fundholding practices in Scotland in 1990 and 1992: needs process and outcome, *British Journal of General Practice*, **45**, 121–6.

Howie, J., Home, J.G., Heaney, D.J., Maxwell, M. *et al.* (1992) The chief scientist reports. The Scottish general practice shadow fundholding project. Outline of an evaluation, *Health Bulletin, Edinburgh*, **50**(4), 316–28.

Hudson, B. (1994) Locality commissioning in health care, *Health and Social Care in the Community*, **2**(6), 373–8.

Hudson, B., Lewis, H., Waddington, E. and Wistow, G. (1998) *Pathways to Partnership. The Interface Between Social Care and Primary Health Care: National Mapping Exercise*, Leeds: Nuffield Institute for Health/Association of Directors of Social Services.

Hughes, G., Mears, R. and Winch, C. (1997) An inspector calls? Regulation and accountability in three public services, *Policy and Politics*, **25**(3), 299–313.

Huntingdon, J. (1993) From FPC to FHSA to… health commission? *British Medical Journal*, **306**, 33–6.

Hutchinson, A., Foy, C. and Sandhu, B. (1989) Comparison of two scores for allocating resources to doctors in deprived areas, *British Medical Journal*, **299**, 142–4.

Illich, I. (1976) *Limits to Medicine*, London: Calder & Boyars.

Illiffe, S. and Haug, U. (1991) Out of hours calls in general practice, *British Medical Journal*, **302**, 1584–6.

Jarman, B. (1981) *A Survey of Primary Care in London*, RCGP Occasional Paper No. 16, London: Royal College of General Practitioners.

Jarman, B. (1983) Identification of underprivileged areas, *British Medical Journal*, **286**, 1705–9.

Jarman, B. (1984) Underprivileged areas: validation and distribution of scores, *British Medical Journal*, **289**, 1587–92.

Jarman, B. (1989) General practice. In A. While (ed.) *Health in the Inner City*, London: Heinemann.

Jarman, B. (1993) Is London overbedded? *British Medical Journal*, **306**, 979–82.

Jarman, B., Bosanquet, N., Rice, P., Dollimore, N. *et al.* (1988) Uptake of immunisation in district health authorities in England, *British Medical Journal*, **296**, 1775–8.

Jenkins, C. and Campbell, J. (1996) Catchment areas in general practice and their relation to size and quality of practice and deprivation: a descriptive study in one London borough, *British Medical Journal*, **313**, 1189–92.

Jessop, B., Bonnett, K., Bromley, S. and Ling, T. (1988) *Thatcherism: A Tale of Two Nations*, Cambridge: Polity Press.

Jessop, E. (1992) Individual morbidity and neighbourhood deprivation in a non-metropolitan area, *Journal of Epidemiology and Community Health*, **46**, 543–6.

Jewson, N. (1976) The disappearance of the sick man from medical cosmology, *Sociology*, **10**, 225–44.

Johnson, T. (1972) *Professions and Power*, London: Routledge.

Jones, A., Bentham, G., Harrison, B.O.W., Jarvis, D. *et al.* (1998) Accessibility and health service utilization for asthma in Norfolk, England, *Journal of Public Health Medicine*, **20**, 312–17.

Jones, K. and Kirby, A. (1982) Provision and well-being: an agenda for public resources research, *Environment and Planning A*, **14**, 297–310.

Jones, K. and Moon, G. (1987) *Health, Disease and Society*, London: Routledge & Kegan Paul.

Jones, K. and Moon, G. (1991) Multilevel assessment of immunisation uptake as a performance measure in general practice, *British Medical Journal*, **303**, 28–31.

Jones, K., Moon, G. and Clegg, A. (1992) Ecological and individual effects in childhood immunisation uptake: a multi-level approach, *Social Science and Medicine*, **33**, 501–8.

Joseph Rowntree Foundation (1994) *Disadvantage in Rural Scotland*, York: Joseph Rowntree Foundation.

Kammerling, R.M. and Kinnear, A. (1996) The extent of the two tier service for fundholders, *British Medical Journal*, **312**, 1399–1401.

Kearns, R. and Barnett, R. (1992) Enter the supermarket: entrepreneurial medical practice in New Zealand, *Environment and Planning C*, **10**, 267–81.

Kearns, R. and Barnett, R. (1997) Consumerist ideology and the symbolic landscapes of private medicine, *Health and Place*, **3**, 171–80.

Kelsey, J. (1995) *The New Zealand Experiment: A World Model for Structural Adjustment*, Auckland: Auckland University Press.

Kelson, M. and Redpath, L. (1996) Promoting user involvement in clinical audit: surveys of audit committees in primary and secondary care, *Journal of Clinical Effectiveness*, **1**, 14–18.

Kendrick, T. and Hilton, S. (1997) Broader teamwork in primary care, *British Medical Journal*, **314**, 672–5.

Kenny, C. (1998) Fury over GP domination of primary care groups, *Nursing Times*, **94**(25), 7.

Khan, P. and Lupton, C. (1999) *Working Together or Pulling Apart*, Portsmouth: Social Services Research and Information Unit, University of Portsmouth.

King's Fund (1992) *London Health Care 2010*, London: King's Fund.

Kirkman-Liff, B. (1997) The United States. In C. Ham (ed.) *Health Care Reform: Learning From International Experience*, Buckingham: Open University Press.

Klazinga, N. (1994) Compliance with practice guidelines: clinical autonomy revisited, *Health Policy*, **28**, 51–66.

Klein, R. (1986) Controlling the gatekeepers: the accountability of general practitioners, *Journal of the Royal College of General Practitioners*, **36**, 129–30.

Klein, R. (1990) From status to contract: the transformation of the British medical profession. In H. L'Etang (ed.) *Health Care Provision Under Financial Constraint: A Decade of Change*, Royal Society of Medicine Services International Congress and Symposium Series No. 171, London: Royal Society of Medicine Services.

Klein, R. (1995) *The New Politics of the NHS*, London: Longman.

Klein, R. (1998) Regulating the medical profession: doctors and the public interest. In A. Harrison (ed.) *Health Care UK 1997/98*, London: King's Fund.

Knox, P. (1978) The intra-urban ecology of primary medical care: patterns of accessibility and their policy implications, *Environment and Planning A*, **10**, 415–35.

Knox, P. (1979) Medical deprivation, area deprivation and public policy, *Social Science and Medicine*, **13D**, 111–21.

Krasnik, A. (1990) Changing remuneration systems: effects on activity in general practices, *British Medical Journal*, **300**, 1698–7701.

Larson, M. (1977) *The Rise of Professionalism: A Sociological Analysis*, Berkeley, CA: University of California Press.

Leavey, R. and Wood, J. (1985) Does the underprivileged area index work? *British Medical Journal*, **291**, 709–11.

Leavey, R., Wilkin, D. and Metcalfe, D. (1989) Consumerism and general practice, *British Medical Journal*, **298**, 737–9.

Leedham, I. and Wistow, G. (1992) *Community Care and General Practitioners*, Working Paper No. 6, Leeds: Nuffield Institute.

Leese, B. and Bosanquet, N. (1992) Immunisation in the UK: policy review and future economic options, *Vaccine*, **10**, 491–9.

Leese, B. and Bosanquet, N. (1995) Change in general practice and its effects on service provision in areas with different socioeconomic characteristics, *British Medical Journal*, **311**, 546–50.

Leese, B. and Bosanquet, N. (1996) Changes in general practice organization: survey of general practitioners' views on the 1990 contract and fundholding, *British Journal of General Practice*, **46**, 95–9.

Le Grand, J. (1998) US managed care: has the UK anything to learn? *British Medical Journal*, **317**, 831–2.

Lewis, G., David, A., Andreasson, S. and Allebeck, P. (1992) Schizophrenia and city life, *Lancet*, **340**, 137–40.

LHPC (London Health Planning Consortium) (1981) *Primary Health Care in Inner London: A Report of a Study Group* (the Acheson London Report); London: DHSS.

Li, J. and Taylor, B. (1991) Comparison of immunisation rates in general practice and child health clinics, *British Medical Journal*, **303**, 1035–8.

Lipsky, M. (1980) *Street Level Bureaucracy: Dilemmas of the Individual in Public Service*, New York: Russell Sage Foundation.

Livingstone, A. and Widgery, D. (1990) The new new general practice: the changing philosophies of primary care, *British Medical Journal*, **301**, 708–10.

Lloyd, P., Lupton, D. and Donaldson, C. (1991) Consumerism in the health care setting: an exploratory study of factors underlying the selection and evaluation of primary medical services, *Australian Journal of Public Health*, **15**(3), 194–201.

Lloyd, D., Harris, C. and Clucas, D. (1995) Low income scheme index: a new deprivation scale based on prescribing in general practice, *British Medical Journal*, **310**, 165–9.

Loudon, I., Horder, J. and Webster, C. (eds) (1998) *General Practice Under the National Health Service 1948–1997*, London: Clarendon Press.

Luft, H. (1994) Health maintenance organisations: is the United States experience applicable to ourselves? In OECD (ed.) *Health Quality and Choice*, Paris: OECD.

Lupton, C., Peckham, S. and Taylor, P. (1998) *Managing Public Involvement in Healthcare Purchasing*, Buckingham: Open University Press.

Lupton, C., Khan, P., North, N. and Lacey, D. (1999) *The Role of Health Professionals in the Child Protection Process*. Portsmouth: Social Services Research and Information Unit, University of Portsmouth.

McCormick, A. Fleming, D. and Charlton, J. (1995) *Morbidity Statistics from General Practice: Results of the Fourth National Study 1991–92*, London: HMSO.

McCulloch, A. and Ashburner, L. (1997) Primary dolours, *Health Service Journal*, **107** (28 August), 22–3.

McIntosh, H., Martin, I. and Wommersley, Y. (1981) Immunisation rates in Glasgow, *Health Bulletin*, March, 92–7.

McIntosh, K. (1999) A word in private, *Health Service Journal*, **109**(5652), 9–11.

McIntyre, K., Miller, J. and Sullivan, F. (1992) The 1990 contract: have patients noticed? *Health Bulletin of Edinburgh*, **50**(1), 7–13.

McKee, C., Gleadhill, D. and Watson, J. (1990) Accident and emergency attendance rates: variation among patients from different general practices, *British Journal of General Practice*, **40**, 150–3.

McKeown, T. (1979) *The Role of Medicine*, Oxford: Blackwell.

McKinlay, J. and Stoekle, J. (1988) Corporatisation and the transformation of doctoring, *International Journal of Health Services*, **18**, 191–205.

McKinstry, B. (1987) Successful liaison between the health team and social workers in Blackburn, West Lothian, *British Medical Journal*, **294** (24 January), 221–4.

McMahon, C. and Bodansky, H. (1991) Attitudes and intentions of UK general practitioners to diabetes care at the time of implementation of their new contract, *Diabetic Medicine*, **8**, 770–2.

Majeed, F., Martin, D. and Crayford, T. (1996) Deprivation payments to general practitioners: limitations of census data, *British Medical Journal*, **313**, 669–70.

Malcolm, L. (1993) Trends in primary medical care related services and expenditure in New Zealand 1983–93, *New Zealand Medical Journal*, **106**, 470–74.

Malcolm, L. and Powell, M. (1996) The development of independent practice associations and related groups in New Zealand, *New Zealand Medical Journal*, **109**, 184–7.

Marks, L. (1987) *Primary Health Care on the Agenda?* London: King's Fund.

Marks, L. (1989) General practice or primary health care? *Journal of Royal College of General Practitioners*, **39**, 1–4.

Marks, L. and Hunter, D. (1998) *The Development of Primary Care Groups: Policy into Practice*, Birmingham: NHS Confederation.

Marsh, G. and Channing, D. (1986) Deprivation and health in one general practice, *British Medical Journal*, **292**, 1173–6.

Maxwell, R. (1993) Other cities, same problems. In J. Smith (ed.) *London After Tomlinson: Reorganising Big City Medicine*, London: BMJ Books.

May, C., Dowrick, C. and Richardson, M. (1996) The confidential patient: the social construction of therapeutic relationships in general practice, *Sociological Review*, **44**, 187–203.

Maynard, A. (1986) Performance incentives in general practice. In G. Teeling-Smith (ed.) *Health Education and General Practice*, London: Office of Health Economics.

Maynard, A. (1997) Evidence-based medicine: an incomplete method for informing treatment choices, *Lancet*, **349**, 126–8.

Mays, N., Goodwin, N., Bevan, G. and Wyke, S. (1997) *Total Purchasing: A Profile of National Pilot Projects*, London: King's Fund.

Mays, N., Goodwin, N., Killoran, A. and Malbon, G. (1998) *Total Purchasing: A Step Towards Primary Care Groups*, London: King's Fund.

Meads, G. (1996) *A Primary Care Led NHS*, London: Churchill Livingstone.

Means, R. and Smith, R. (1994) *Community Care. Policy and Practice*, Basingstoke: Macmillan.

Mechanic, D. (1975) The organization of medical practice and practice orientations among physicians in prepaid and non-prepaid primary care settings, *Medical Care*, **13**, 189–204.

Ministry of Health (1963) *The Field of Work of the Family Doctor*, (The Gillie Report), London: HMSO.

Mohan, J. (1995) Privatisation in the British health service: a challenge to the NHS. In J. Gabe, M. Calnan and M. Bury (eds) *The Sociology of the Health Service*, London: Routledge.

Moore, A. (1995) Deprivation payments in general practice: some spatial issues in resource allocation in the UK, *Health and Place*, **1**, 121–5.

Morley, V., Evans, T., Higgs, R., Lock, P., Allsop, J. (1981) *A Case Study in Developing Primary Care*, London: King's Fund.

Morrell, D. (1989) The new general practitioner contract, *British Medical Journal*, **298**, 1005–7.

Morrell, D., Gage, H. and Robinson, N. (1971) Symptoms in general practice, *Journal of Royal College of General Practitioners*, **21**, 32–43.

Morris, J., Cook, D., Walker, M. and Shaper, A. (1992) Non-consulters and high consulters in general practice: cardio-respiratory health and risk factors, *Journal of Public Health Medicine*, **14**, 131–7.

Morris, R. (1993) Community care and the fundholder, *British Medical Journal*, **306**, 635–6.

MPC (Medical Practices Committee) (1998) *Medical Practices Committee: Annual Report for 1997/1998*, London: MPC.

Munro, J., Nicholl, J., O'Cathain, A. and Knowles, E. (1998) *Evaluation of NHS Direct First Wave Sites. First Interim Report to the Department of Health.* Sheffield: Medical Care Research Unit, University of Sheffield.

Murphy, A., McCafferty, D., Dowling, J. and Bury, G. (1996) One-year prospective study of cases of suspected acute myocardial infarction managed by urban and rural general practitioners, *British Journal of General Practice*, **46**, 73–6.

Myles, S. Wyke, S., Popay, J., Scott, J., Campbell, A. and Girling, J. (1998) *Total Purchasing and Community and Continuing Care: Lessons for Future Policy Developments in the NHS*, London: King's Fund.

NAO (National Audit Office) (1987) *Community Care Developments: Report to the Comptroller and Auditor General*, London: HMSO.

NAO (National Audit Office) (1988) *The Management of Family Practitioner Services*, London: HMSO.

Neal, R.D., Heywood, P.L., Morley, S., Clayden, A.D. *et al.* (1998) Frequency of patients' consulting in general practice and workload generated by frequent attenders: comparisons between practices, *British Journal of General Practice*, **48**, 895–8.

Neve, H. and Taylor, P. (1995) Working with the community, *British Medical Journal*, **311**, 524–5.

New, S. and Senior, M. (1992) 'I don't believe in needles': qualitative aspects of a study into the uptake of infant immunisation in two English health authorities, *Social Science and Medicine*, **33**, 509–18.

Newlands, M. and Davies, L. (1988) The use of performance indicators for immunisation rates in general practice, *Public Health*, **102**, 269–73.

Newton, J. (1996) Patients' involvement in medical audit in general practice, *Health and Social Care in the Community*, **4**(3), 142–9.

NHSE (NHS Executive) (1993) *Better Living – Better Lives*, Leeds: NHSE.

NHSE (NHS Executive) (1994a) *Towards a Primary Care Led NHS: An Accountability Framework for GP Fundholding*, EL(94)92, London: HMSO.

NHSE (NHS Executive) (1994b) *Developing NHS Purchasing and GP Fundholding – Towards a Primary Care-led NHS*, Leeds: NHS Executive.

NHSE (NHS Executive) (1997) *Percentage Coverage of GP Fundholding England 1991/2 and 1996/7; Number of GP Fundholders, Practices and Funds 1991/2 and 1996/7*, Leeds: NHSE.

NHSE (NHS Executive) (1998) *Better Health and Better Health Care. Implementing 'The New NHS' and 'Our Healthier Nation'*, HSC 1998/021, Leeds: NHS Executive.

NHSE General Medical Census Additional Data collection (1994/95 and 1995/96).

NHSME (NHS Management Executive) (1991a) *Purchasing for Health*, Conference Report, London: DoH.

NHSME (NHS Management Executive) (1991b) *Assessing Health Care Needs*, London: DoH.

NHSME (NHS Management Executive) (1991c) *Moving Forward – Needs Services and Contracts*, London: DoH.

NHSME (NHS Management Executive) (1992a) *Local Voices. The Views of Local People in Purchasing for Health*, London: NHSME.

NHSME (NHS Management Executive) (1992b) *The Patient's Charter and Primary Health Care* EL(92)88, London: DoH.

Niskanen, W. (1971) *Bureaucracy and Representative Government*, Chicago: Aldine Atherton.

Noakes, J. (1991) Patients not seen in three years: will invitations for health checks be of benefit? *British Journal of General Practice*, **41**, 335–8.

Nocon, A. (1993) Fair Assessment, *Health Service Journal*, 1 July, 29.

North, N. (1997a) Implementing strategy: the politics of healthcare commissioning, *Policy and Politics*, **26**(1), 5–14.

North, N. (1997b) Politics and procedures: the strategy process in health commission, *Health and Social Care in the Community*, **5**, 375–83.

North, N. (1998) Issues and debates: a new NHS? *Research, Policy and Planning*, **16**(1), 28–32.

North, N., Lupton, C. and Khan, P. (1999) Going with the grain? GPs and the new NHS, *Health and Social Care in the Community*, **7**(6), 409–17.

OHE (Office for Health Economics) (1966) *General Practice Today*, London: OHE.

OHE (Office for Health Economics) (1995) *Compendium of Statistics*, 9th edn, London: OHE.

OHE (Office for Health Economics) (1997) *Compendium of Statistics*, 10th edn, London: OHE.

Okma, K. (1995) Restructuring health care in the Netherlands. In R. Williams (ed.) *International Developments in Health Care: A Review of Health Care Systems in the 1990s*, London: Royal College of Physicians.

Oldham, J. and Rutter, I. (1999) Independence days, *British Medical Journal*, **318**, 748–9.

ONS (Office for National Statistics) (1995) *The General Household Survey*, London: HMSO.

O'Reilly, D. and Steele, K. (1998) More equitable systems for allocating general practice deprivation payments: financial consequences, *British Journal of General Practice*, **48**, 1405–7.

Ottewill, R. and Wall, A. (1990) *The Growth and Development of the Community Health Services*, Sunderland: Business Education Publishers.

Øvretveit, J. (1995) *Purchasing for Health*, Buckingham: Open University Press.

Panel of Inquiry (1989) *Tyra Henry: Whose Child? The Report of the Panel Appointed To Inquire into the Death of Tyra Henry*, London: Lambeth Borough Council.

Paris, J., Wakeman, A. and Griffiths, R. (1992) General practitioners and public health, *Public Health*, **106**, 357–66.

Parkhouse, J. (1991) *Doctors' Careers: Aims and Experiences of Medical Graduates*, London: Routledge.

Parry, N. and Parry, J. (1976) *The Rise of the Medical Profession*, London: Croom Helm.

Peckham, C. (1989) *National Immunisation Study: Factors Influencing Immunisation Uptake in Childhood*, London: Institute for Child Health.

Pedersen, L. and Leese, B. (1997) What will a primary care led NHS mean for GP workload? The problem of the lack of an evidence base, *British Medical Journal*, **314**, 1337–41.

PEP (Political and Economic Planning (1944) *Medical Care for Citizens*, Broadsheet 222, London: PEP.

Pereira Gray, D. (1994) Twenty-five years of development in general practice, *Health Trends*, **26**(1), 4–5.

Pereira Gray, D., Marinker, M. and Maynard, A. (1986) The doctor, the patient, and their contract, *British Medical Journal*, **292**, 1313–15.

Perkins, E. (1991) Screening elderly people: a review of the literature in the light of the new general practitioner contract, *British Journal of General Practice*, **41**, 382–5.

Petchey, R. (1987) Health maintenance organisations: just what the doctor ordered? *Journal of Social Policy*, **16**, 489–507.

Petchey, R. (1995) Collings' report on general practice in England in 1950: unrecognised, pioneering piece of British social research? *British Medical Journal*, **311**, 40–2.

Petchey, R. (1996) From stableboys to jockeys? The prospects for a primary care-led NHS. In J. Baldcock and M. May (eds) *Social Policy Review 8*, Kent: Social Policy Association.

Phillimore, P. and Reading, R. (1992) A rural advantage? Urban–rural health differences in Northern England, *Journal of Public Health Medicine*, **14**, 290–9.

Pietroni, P. and Chase, H. (1993) Patients or partisans? Patient participation at Marylebone Health Centre, *British Journal of General Practice*, **43**, 341–4.

Pollitt, C., Harrison, S., Hunter, D., and Marnoch, G. (1991) General management in the NHS: the initial impact, 1983–88, *Public Administration*, **69** (Spring), 61–83.

Porter, R. (1999) And how are the GPs doing? *Times Higher Education Supplement*, 8 January, 29.

Powell, M. (1987) Access to Primary Health Care in London. Unpublished PhD thesis, London: University of London.

Powell, M. (1990) Need for and provision of general practice in London, *British Journal of General Practice*, **40**, 372–5.

Powell, M. (1992) A tale of two cities: a critical evaluation of the geographical provision of health care before the NHS, *Public Administration*, **70**, 67–80.

Powell, M. (1995) A geographical analysis of the distribution of doctors in 1938. Paper presented to the Quantitative Economic and Social History Conference, St Catherine's College, University of Cambridge.

Powell, M. (1997) *Evaluating the National Health Service*, Milton Keynes: Open University Press.

Poxton, R. (1994) *Joint Commissioning: The Story So Far*, Briefing No. 1, Joint Community Care Commissioning Project, London: King's Fund.

Pratt, J. (1995) *Practitioners and Practices*, Oxford: Radcliffe Medical Press.

Pringle, M. (1999) Letters, *Independent*, 19 June.

Pringle, M. and Heath, I. (1997) Primary care: opportunities and threats, *British Medical Journal*, **314**, 595.

Pringle, M. and Morton-Jones, A. (1994) Using unemployment rates to predict prescribing trends in England, *British Journal of General Practice*, **44**, 53–6.

Raffel, M. and Raffel, N. (1994) *The US Health System*, Albany: Delmar.

Raistrick, S. (1988) Free health care – at a price, *British Medical Journal*, **297**, 47–9.

Ranade, W. (1997) *A Future for the NHS? Health Care for the Millennium*, London: Longman.

Rawles, J., Sinclair, C., Jennings, K., Ritchie, L. *et al.* (1998) Call to needle times after acute myocardial infarction in urban and rural areas in north-east Scotland: prospective observational study, *British Medical Journal*, **317**, 576–8.

RCGP (Royal College of General Practitioners) (1985) *Quality in General Practice*, London: RCGP.

RCGP (Royal College of General Practitioners) (1987) *The Front Line of the Health Service: The College Response to 'Primary Health Care – An Agenda for Discussion'*, London: RCGP.

RCGP (Royal College of General Practitioners) (1996) *The Nature of General Practice*, Report No. 27, London: RCGP.

RCGP (Royal College of General Practitioners) (1998) *Inner City General Practice: A Factsheet*, London: RCGP.

RDC (Rural Development Commission) (1998) *1997 Survey of Rural Services*, Salisbury: RDC.

Reading, R., Raybould, S. and Jarvis, S. (1993) Deprivation, low birth weight and children's height, *British Medical Journal*, **307**, 1458–62.

Rice, T. (1983) The impact of changing Medicare reimbursement rates on physician-induced demand, *Medical Care*, **21**, 803–15.

Richards, J., Jacoby, A. and Bone, M. (1981) *Access to Primary Care*, London: HMSO.

Rimmer, B. and Ross, S. (1997) Perspectives on primary care prescribing, *Health Bulletin*, **55**(4), 243–61.

Ritchie, L., Bisset, A., Russell, D., Leslie,V. and Thomson, I. (1992) Primary and preschool immunisation in Grampian: progress and the 1990 contract, *British Medical Journal*, **304**, 816–19.

Robinson, R. (1998) Managed competition: health care reform in the Netherlands. In W. Ranade (ed.) *Markets and Health Care: A Comparative Analysis*, London: Longman.

Robinson, R. and Hayter, P. *Why GPs Choose Not to Apply as Fundholders*. Southampton: IHPS, University of Southampton.

Robinson, R. and Steiner, A. (1998) *Managed Health Care*, Buckingham: Open University Press.

Rogers, A., Hassell, K. and Nicolaas, G. (1999) *Demanding Patients? Analysing the Use of Primary Health Care*, London: Open University Press.

Rosen, B. (1989) Professional reimbursement and professional behaviour: emerging issues and research challenges, *Social Science and Medicine*, **29**(3), 455–67.

Royal Commission on the NHS (1979) *The Report of the Royal Commission on the NHS*, London: HMSO.

Ryan, M. and Yule, B. (1993) The way to economic prescribing, *Health Policy*, **25**, 25–38.

Salisbury, C. (1989) How do people choose their doctor? *British Medical Journal*, **299**, 608–10.

Salmon, J. (1985) Profit and health care: trends in corporatization and proprietization, *International Journal of Health Services*, **15**, 395–418.

Schut, F. and Van Doorslaer, E. (1999) Towards a reinforced agency role of health insurers in Belgium and the Netherlands, *Health Policy*, **48**, 47–67.

Scottish Consumer Council (1997) *Scoping Study on Patient Involvement in Primary Care in Scotland*, Edinburgh: Scottish Consumer Council.

Scottish Office Department of Health (1997) *Designed to Care. Renewing the National Health Service in Scotland*, Cm 3811, Edinburgh: DoH.

Scottish Office Department of Health (1998) *NHS Complaints in Scotland, 1997/8*, Statistical Bulletin 1/98, Edinburgh: DoH.

Scott-Samuel, A. (1984) Need for primary health care: an objective indicator, *British Medical Journal*, **288**, 457–8.

Seivewright, H., Tyrer, P., Casey, P. and Seivewright, N. (1991) A three-year follow-up of psychiatric morbidity in urban and rural primary care, *Psychological Medicine*, **21**, 495–503.

Senior, M. (1991) Deprivation payments to GPs: not what the doctor ordered, *Environment and Planning C*, **9**, 79–94.

Senior, M. (1995) Updating or radically changing deprivation payments to GPs in England: experiments using 1991 census data. Paper presented the Institute of British Geographers Annual Conference, University of Northumbria, Newcastle upon Tyne.

Shackley, P. and Ryan, M. (1994) What is the role of the consumer in health care? *Journal of Social Policy*, **23**(4), 517–41.

Sheppard, M. (1992) Contact and collaboration with general practitioners: a comparison of social workers and community nurses, *British Journal of Social Work*, **22**, 419–36.

Shucksmith, M., Roberts, D., Scott, D., Chapman, P. and Conway, E. (1996) *Disadvantage in Rural Areas*, Salisbury: Rural Development Commission.

Silagy, C. and Haines, A. (1998) *Evidence-based Practice in Primary Care*, London: BMJ Books.

Smith, C. and Armstrong, D. (1989) Comparison of criteria derived by government and patients for evaluating general practitioner services, *British Medical Journal*, **299**, 494–6.

Smith, J. and Shapiro, J. (1997) Local call, *Health Service Journal*, **107**(5535), 26–7.

Smith, J., Bamford, M., Ham, C. and Shapiro, J. (1997) *Beyond Fundholding: A Mosaic of Primary Care Led Commissioning and Provision in the West Midlands*, Health Services Management Centre, University of Birmingham /Centre for Health Planning and Management, Keele University.

Smith, R. (1998) All changed, changed utterly, *British Medical Journal*, **313**, 18.

Social Services Committee (1985) *Second Report from the Social Services Committee, Community Care with Special Reference to Adult Mentally Ill and Mentally Handicapped People*, London: HMSO.

Spurgeon, P., Barwell, F. and Maxwell, R. (1995) Types of work stress and implications for the role of general practitioners, *Health Services Management Research*, **8**(3), 186–97.

Stacey, M. (1992) *Regulating British Medicine*, Chichester: John Wiley & Sons.

Starfield, B. (1997) The future of primary care in a managed care era, *International Journal of Health Services*, **27**(4), 687–96.

Stevens, R. (1966) *Medical Practice in Modern England*, London: Yale University Press.

Stewart-Brown, S., Surender, R., Bradlow, J., Coulter, A. *et al.* (1995) The effects of fundholding in general practice on prescribing habits three years after introduction of the scheme, *British Medical Journal*, **311**, 1543–7.

Stilwell, B. (1991) The rise of the practice nurse, *Nursing Times*, **87**(24), 26–8.

Strong, P. and Robinson, J. (1990) *The NHS Under New Management*, Milton Keynes: Open University Press.

Surender, R., Bradlow, J., Coulter, A., Doll, H. and Stewart Brown, S. (1995) Prospective study of trends in referral patters in fundholding and non-fundholding practices in the Oxford region, 1990–4, *British Medical Journal*, **311**, 1205–8.

Thomas, K., Nicholl, J. and Coleman, P. (1995) Assessing the outcome of making it easier for patients to change general practitioner: practice characteristics associated with patient movements, *British Journal of General Practice*, **45**, 581–6.

Thomas, R. and Corney, R. (1992) A survey of links between mental health professionals and general practice in six district health authorities, *British Journal of General Practice*, **42**, 368–81.

Thomas, R. and Corney, R. (1993) Working together with community mental health professionals: a survey among general practitioners, *British Journal of General Practice*, **43**(October), 417–21.

Thompson, N. (1990) Inviting infrequent attenders to attend for a health check: costs and benefits, *British Journal of General Practice*, **40**, 16–18.

Timmins, N. (1988) *Cash Crisis and Cure: The Independent Guide to the NHS Debate*, London: Newspaper Publishing.

Timmins, N. (1995) *The Five Giants: A Biography of the Welfare State*, London: HarperCollins.

Titmuss, R. (1963) *Essays on the Welfare State*, London: Unwin.

Tudor Hart, J. (1971) The inverse care law, *Lancet*, 27 February, 405–12.

Tudor Hart, J. (1988) *A New Kind of Doctor*, London: Merlin Press.

Tudor Hart, J. (1995) Clinical and economic consequences of patients as producers, *Journal of Public Health Medicine*, **17**(4), 383–6.

Tudor Hart, M. (1981) A new kind of doctor, *Journal of the Royal Society of Medicine*, **74**, 871–83.

Turnberg, L. (1998) *Health Services in London: A Strategic Review*, London: HMSO.

Twigg, J. and Atkin, K. (1995) Carers and services: factors dictating service provision, *Journal of Social Policy*, **24**(1), 5–30.

van de Ven, W. (1997) The Netherlands. In C. Ham (ed.) *Health Care Reform: Learning From International Experience*, Buckingham: Open University Press.

van de Ven, W. and Rutten, F. (1994) Managed competition in the Netherlands: lessons from five years of health reform, *Australian Health Review*, **17**(3), 9–27.

van de Ven, W. and Schut, F. (1995) The Dutch experience with internal markets. In M. Jerome-Forget, J. White and J. Wiener (eds) *Health Reform Through Internal Markets: Experience and Proposals*, Montreal: Institute for Research on Public Policy.

van de Ven, W., Vanvliet, R.C.J.A., Vanbarneveld, E.M. and Larners, L.M. (1994) Risk-adjusted capitation: recent experiences in the Netherlands, *Health Affairs*, **13**, 130–6.

Wallace, H. and Mulcahy, L. (1999) *Cause for Complaint? An Evaluation of the Effectiveness of the NHS Complaints Procedure*, Public Law Project, London: Birkbeck College, University of London.

Walker, A. and Rees, L. (1985) Mythical contraindications to vaccination, *Lancet*, **1**(8345), 994.

Waller, D., Agass, M., Mant, D., Coulter, A. *et al.* (1990) Health checks in general practice: another example of inverse care, *British Medical Journal*, **300**, 1115–18.

Ward, P., Huddy, J., Hargreaves, S., Touquet, R. *et al.* (1996) Primary care in London: an evaluation of general practitioners working in an inner city accident and emergency department, *Journal of Accident and Emergency Medicine*, **13**, 11–15.

Watt, G. (1996) All together now: why social deprivation matters, *British Medical Journal*, **312**, 1026–9.

Webb, A. and Wistow, G. (1986) *Planning, Need and Scarcity: Essays on the Personal Social Services*, London: Allen & Unwin.

Webster, C. (1988) *The Health Services since the War*. Vol. I, *Problems of Health Care. The National Health Service before 1957*, London: HMSO.

Webster, C. (1996) *The Health Services since the War*, Vol. II, *Government and Health Care. The National Health Service 1958–1979*, London: HMSO.

Weiner, J. and De Lissovoy, G. (1993) Razing a tower of Babel: a taxonomy for managed care and health insurance plans, *Journal of Health Politics, Policy and Law*, **18**, 75–103.

Welsh Office (1998a) *Health Statistics Wales*, Cardiff: Welsh Office.

Welsh Office (1998b) *NHS Wales: Putting Patients First*, Cm 3841, Cardiff: Welsh Office.

West, M. and Field, R. (1995) Teamwork in primary health care, 1: perspectives from organisational psychology, *Journal of Interprofessional Care*, **9**(2), 117–22.

West, M. and Poulton, B. (1997) A failure of function: teamwork in primary health care, *Journal of Interprofessional Care*, **11**(20), 205–16.

Whitehead, M. (1994) Who cares about equity in the NHS? *British Medical Journal*, **308**, 1284–7.

Whitehouse, C. (1985) Effect of distance from surgery on consultation rates in an urban practice, *British Medical Journal*, **290**, 359–62.

WHO (World Health Organization) (1978) *Primary Health Care: Report of an International Conference on Primary Health Care, Alma Ata*, Geneva: WHO.

Widgery, D. (1991) *Some Lives: A GP's East End*, London: Sinclair Stevenson.

Wiles, R. and Robison, J. (1994) Teamwork in primary care: the views and experiences of nurses, midwives and health visitors, *Journal of Advanced Nursing*, **20**, 324–30.

Wilkin, D. and Metcalfe, D. (1984) List size and patient contact in general medical practice, *British Medical Journal*, **289**, 1501–5.

Wilkin, D., Hallam, L., Leavey, R. and Metcalfe, D. (1987) *The Anatomy of Urban General Practice*, London: Tavistock.

Willcocks, A. (1967) *The Creation of the National Health Service*, London: Routledge & Kegan Paul.

Williams, S. and Calnan, M. (1991) Key determinants of consumer satisfaction with general practice, *Family Practice*, **8**, 237–42.

Williams, S., Calnan, M., Cant, S. and Coyle, J. (1993) All change in the NHS? Implications of the NHS reforms for primary care prevention, *Sociology of Health and Illness*, **15**, 43–67.

Williamson, C. (1999) The challenge of lay partnership, *British Medical Journal*, **319**, 721–2.

Willis, A. (1996) Commissioning – the best for all. In P. Littlejohns and C. Victor (eds) *Making Sense of a Primary Care-led Health Service*, Oxford: Radcliffe Medical Press.

Wistow, G. (1995) Aspirations and realities: community care at the crossroads, *Health and Social Care in the Community*, **3**(4), 227–40.

Wood, J. (1983) Are the problems of primary care in inner cities fact or fiction? *British Medical Journal*, **286**, 1109–12.

Wood, N., Wilkinson, C. and Kumar, A. (1997) Do the homeless get a fair deal from general practitioners? *Journal of the Royal Society of Health*, **117**, 292–7.

Worrall, A., Rea, J. and Ben-Shlomo, Y. (1997) Counting the cost of social disadvantage in primary care: retrospective analysis of patient data, *British Medical Journal*, **314**, 38–42.

Wyke, S., Campbell, G. and Maciver, S. (1992) Provision of and patient satisfaction with primary care services in a relatively affluent area and a relatively deprived area of Glasgow, *British Journal of General Practice*, **42**, 271–5.

Yen, L. (1995) From Alma Ata to Asda and beyond: a commentary on the transition in health promotion services in primary care from commodity to control. In R. Bunton, S. Nettleton and R. Burrows (eds) *The Sociology of Health Promotion: Critical Analyses of Consumption, Lifestyle and Risk*, London: Routledge.

Index

Page numbers printed in **bold** type refer to figures; those in *italic* to tables; a letter n following a page number denotes a note number on that page.